Letters To The Big C

Chris Sypolt

Samothrace Enterprises, LLC
Seattle, WA

ISBN-13: 978-0615902975
ISBN-10: 0615902979

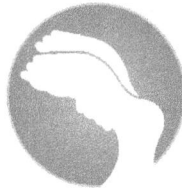

SAMOTHRACE ENTERPRISES

For Carla, who showed me how to dance on the lawn under the eternal blue sky one summer evening in Seattle.

Well she was an American girl
Raised on promises
She couldn't help thinkin'
That there was a little more to life
somewhere else
- "American Girl", Tom Petty

Celebrate we will
Because life is short but sweet for certain
We're climbing two by two
To be sure these days continue
These things we cannot change
- "Two Step", Dave Matthews Band

And when that fog horn blows I will be
coming home
And when the fog horn blows I want to hear
it
I don't have to fear it

And I want to rock your gypsy soul
Just like way back in the days of old
And magnificently we will flow into the
mystic
- "Into The Mystic", Van Morrison

Table of Contents

5

7

In The Beginning, There Were The Text Messages...

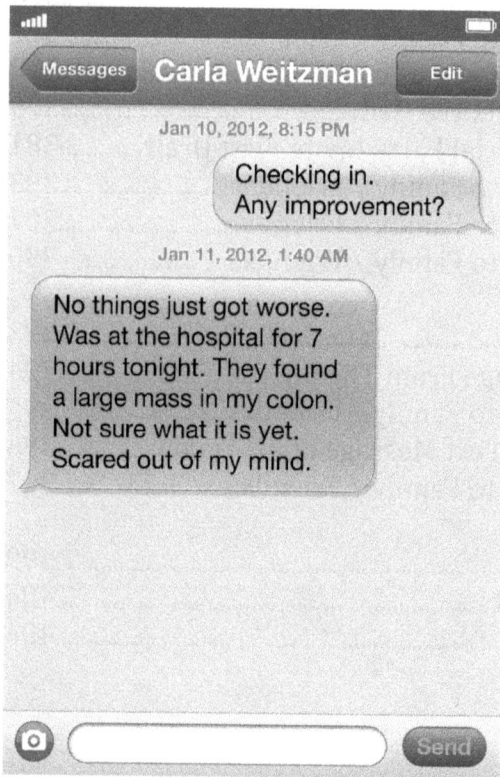

Jan 10, 2012, 8:15 PM

Checking in.
Any improvement?

Jan 11, 2012, 1:40 AM

No things just got worse.
Was at the hospital for 7
hours tonight. They found
a large mass in my colon.
Not sure what it is yet.
Scared out of my mind.

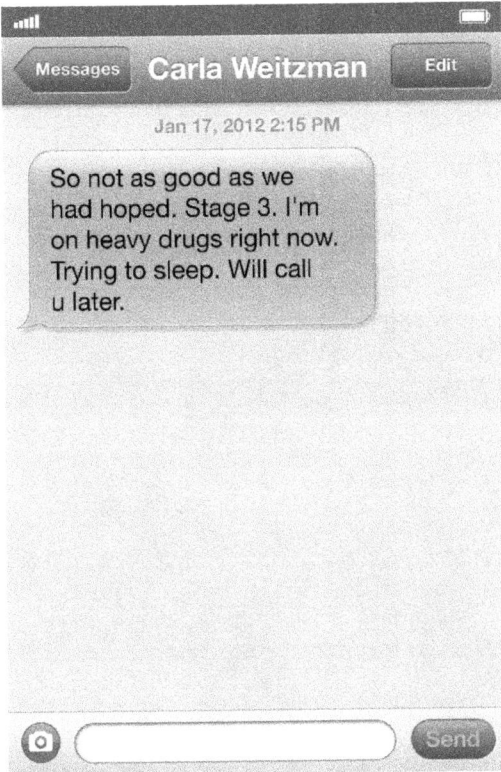

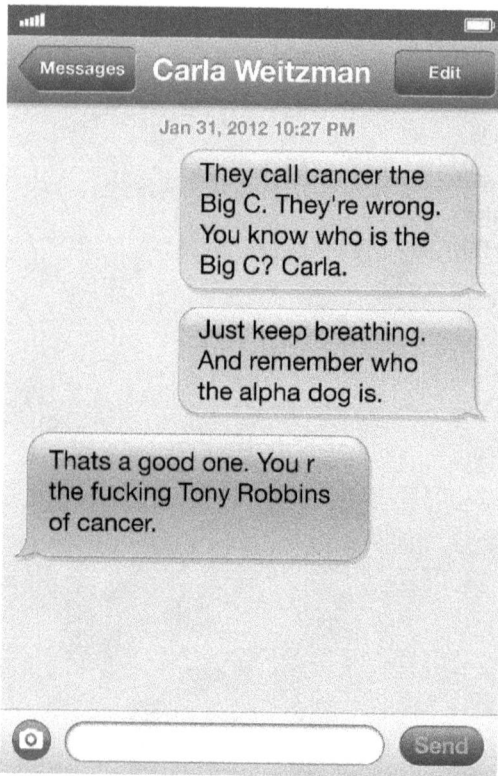

At least the secret about the name of the book is out.

Foreword

Letters To The Big C is both a war story and a love story. It is built from the emailed letters from my friend, Chris Sypolt, to his best friend, Carla Weitzman, who is fighting for her life against the invisible and invasive enemy of colon cancer. Chris sent these letters to Carla mostly in the dark of night, so if she woke, as the world slept, she would never feel alone or weary in combat. He occupied Carla's struggle, he moved in with it, and he brought everything and every part of his being with him. He wasn't leaving in a day or two, or next week, or in 6 months. He stayed as though he liked that place of sickness and suffering and fear, because she was there, and he could ease her pain.

I have paid the dues of cancer. I am fully aware of Carla's struggle, and I see, from a unique vantage point, the value of this work. I am simultaneously awed and astonished by my friend, Chris, and his dedication to his best friend. He props her up with his words. She recognizes that he will be there and she sees him returning again, again, always, and again. Carla knows that Chris will not leave her on the battlefield, damaged, alone, and shaken. He makes certain Carla never has to face the most fearful impossibilities of treatment with no one there. He holds her heart and her soul and, as a result, he nurtures her ability to fabricate a full suit of armor, her protection in the dispute with the opposing force. He makes her worthy of the road and mostly fearless in her attack. The letters dress Carla in courageous armament. The painful and sadistic jabbing, and stabbing, and poison, and burning, of life with cancer are suddenly not what they might have been.

My diagnosis of lung cancer came in mid-November 2009. News of that nature changes a person in ways a human being does not deserve to be changed. For me, it began a period of darkness and fear, complete with automatic

13

initiation into a world sustained by the unfamiliar, and propagated by the emptiness of uncertainty. Cancer, like all terminal or chronically debilitating disease, is a first-class ticket to anxiety, and pain, and pessimism, no matter what you may have thought about it before you became so personally fused to it. And then there are all the other unsuspecting passengers it gathers up and assigns seats to, on what is your trip into the abyss. Cancer is never satisfied with just a single traveler.

Worry quickly becomes the place where you dwell, your new focus when you wake, and your last thought when you close your eyes in ridiculous and exhaustive attempts to sleep. Where will you find the necessary level of support, inspiration, and love? Where do you look for an answer of that magnitude? How do you make peace with a level of threat that shuts down the most famously brilliant, those destined for sainthood, and even the wealthiest among us who can afford the best in treatment and care? Can you turn to your faith and have it speak patience and promise at the volume you need it prayed? Are you able to depend on the medical professionals to sacrifice their time with the next patient, and the next, and the next, and the next, so that you can bleed your worry and endless questioning out on the exam room floor each visit? Do you additionally burden those you love the most, who are also filled with fear, with the screaming that is in your head and clamors to be let out? Where do you turn at 3 AM when you are awake and frightened and choking on tears and aversion and loathing?

I had clear and uncompromising resources supporting my struggle each and every day. Combined, they were a solid force of attendants, companions, gurus, and guides. I am grateful for every one of them and the endless effort they extended on my behalf. They got me through the war, but I couldn't bring myself to ask them for the habitual daily infusion of optimism and inspiration I truly needed to fight my best fight. I couldn't ask any one of them for Carla's armor, or late-night letters. They were already worn from the war and I needed them to keep fighting, at any level. The biggest falsehood related to supporting a patient or the self-support that comes from within the patient, is that it is enough to stare down debilitating disease. It is not enough.

I searched for material that would fortify my soul, lift my spirit, and lead me to a new way of thinking about cancer, one that would offer strategies for feeling less alone with it. I consulted my oncologist, the Internet, every bit of published information I could find, books, and other cancer survivors. There was little to be found that was useful for my battered psyche yet pleasant and hopeful, and engaging to read. I searched for a manual on coping, one that told a bigger story and showed me there can be joy and blessing in cancer. I was looking for Carla's armor. I didn't find it. It wasn't out there then. It is now.

There is remarkable assistance to be found in Letters To The Big C, for the patient and caregiver alike. Anyone who faces the weakening of their body and spirit, or the mental and physical hardship of treatment for any chronic condition, needs alignment with the forces that fill this book. It's a story of two friends, one trying the only way he knows how to save the other, and is filled with soldiering, hope and grace, fight and steadying, pop culture references of inspiration, and the perfect mix of humor. It is fortitude and bolstering, a flight of words to the essence of brave, served up on a chronological path of emailed letters to a place of comfort. It's the positive and persistent energy required to meet the rigors and judgments of cancer and the manifestations of all debilitating diseases. It is unconditional love in its purest form and all the light and air that those who suffer don't know where to find or how to ask for. It's the new and excellent member of the team, encouraging and invigorating the network, it eases the strain, and strengthens and extends foundations.

After surgery to remove my right lung, followed by 3 months of chemotherapy, my cancer has remained in remission for almost 4 years. The continued diagnosis is filled with expectations of good health. I keep gathered all the optimism of Letters To The Big C and, on behalf of all of us, I thank Chris for sharing his inspirations, and for my renewal to promise, and peace, and positivity because he did. His words speak to everyone's future with cancer. His effort saves us from being afraid. Letters To The Big C wasn't written for me but it makes me fearless. It is the joy, the blessing, and the gift of cancer.

Mary Ann Evans
Cancer Survivor
Kingston, New York

Prologue

For a large portion of 2012, my best friend, Carla Weitzman, was locked in a battle for her life. In her case, it was colon cancer, incredibly rare in those under 50, and with no family history. She had a large team of friends to support her and to help with the day-to-day logistical tasks she needed help with. I played my part as well in that role.

But I also had a different role. Beginning very early on in her treatment, I sent her an email. Every night. I was in some ways uniquely qualified to do this for her – I'd been emailing her long 4,000-word rants for years, typed out on, of all things, a Blackberry (I later saw the error of my ways and switched to the iPhone). She would read them on her ride into work and laugh her ass off and then call me when she got into the office and tell me what I was wrong about.

These emails were different – rather than ranting about business or politics or religion, these were about keeping her motivated, about trying to help her realize how loved she was, about inspiring her. And about keeping the 3 AM wolves away.

There is a time, in the middle of the night, when very few people are awake. Generally speaking, those people either have the night shift, or they are cancer patients. The second group is worried, anxious, and fearful. They don't really know what's happening to them, because the medical industry sucks, or they have a good idea, and they're frightened and alone, even with a partner sleeping soundly beside them.

This book is dedicated to each of you who are having 3 am moments. You're not alone. As my dad, The Fox (who you will see more of along the way) used to say – "At least a billion people have done this before you". This doesn't take away the worry or the fear, but it reminds you that others have walked down this path. More and more win their fight every day. It is neither fair nor right that you are here, but you are.

This is also dedicated to the caretakers. Hopefully, it is the first and only time that you will have to be in this position, helping your friend or loved one to confront the unspeakable. It is, for sure, not a club that you want to be a member of, but you are now. If you think the initiation rites were bad, wait until it comes time to pay the dues. You are the protectors. You will never be thanked as much as you probably should be, but if you're doing it for thanks, you're doing it for the wrong reason.

There is an obvious tendency to dwell on the hard parts, because they are hard. But it doesn't have to be that way. I found myself celebrating victories, small and large, all along the way. And I found a way to openly express my love for my best friend. The times when we were alone and I was taking care of her are something that I will remember forever. I felt that I was in exactly the right place at exactly the right time.

Letters To The Big C is an extension of that feeling. I've always been fortunate in that I can put the nouns and verbs in the right order, and my typos are so rare that in 13 years at my previous company, only a single one was found.

This book is all of the emails (minus a couple of absolutely inane entries) that I sent to Carla during her fight. In some places it is raw inspiration, in some part a simple chronicle of events. Above all, the letters helped keep the 3 AM wolves at bay – the emails would arrive at midnight or 1 AM, typically after I had had a couple of drinks, and if Carla had a bad night, she could be assured of seeing something new to help her carry the burden.

I have some very specific spiritual beliefs and convictions, but God/Buddha/YHWH/Allah/The Force does not need me to market these things. Some of them come out along the way (that's part of the story as well), but this is not about spirituality or belief in a certain set of defined principles or tenets. I know from personal experience that it helps to be aware of these things and practice them, but that is as far as I'll go – choose the things that work for you, because they're likely all coming from the same source.

Now, while I'm not going to advocate any specific spiritual approach, I am going to advocate trying to tap into something, anything, that allows you to Believe more deeply. Believe that you will recover. Believe that your partner and your kids will be OK. Believe that you've been given a great gift. Believe in the power of love and grace and belief. Because it is there, and as difficult as it is to understand, you'll never be closer to those things than you are now.

When Carla was first diagnosed, I did what any good geek would do - I went looking for a manual about what to do and what not to do for my friend. I really couldn't find one. I joined a support group (albeit for two weeks, because every person in there had a family member who was dying, and Carla's prognosis was overwhelmingly positive). I really didn't know how to act. Carla was the first person in my peer group to be affected by something life-threatening.

But I did know how to write. For years, I'd gotten a buzz on at the local watering hole and produced, in Carla's words, "these 4,000 word rants put together on an iPhone WITH NO TYPOS OR GRAMMATICAL ERRORS."

Sometimes they were germane to something that was going on between the two of us, but most of the time I would see something stupid on the news or at work that I felt the need to comment on. She'd get them in the morning during her bus ride, and whether she agreed or not, she enjoyed the rants for what they were.

A brief word about our interactions - while Carla was born and raised in Seattle, her soul is that of someone raised on the East Coast. She never has a problem confronting people on their bullshit, which is pretty much the opposite of the stereotypical native Seattleite. We got along from the first moment that we met at a business function in 1999.

For whatever reason, we clicked. We could argue pop culture, or politics, or history, or whatever subject was on the table. We would do so in the most vociferous way possible - friends of ours refused to watch, it appeared so vicious from the outside. But every single time, when we were done, we always ask each other - "was it good for you?" And it always is. There are never any hard feelings. It is special. It is cathartic. It is an honest exchange of views between two close friends.

We did date for a couple of months in 1999, but broke up because we were far better friends than lovers. I was responsible, in a way, for her meeting the man who became her husband. I also ended up being the best man and maid of honor in 2003 when Stu and Carla eloped to Las Vegas, and was honored to fill that role for them. I have to hand it to Stu - he always understood how close she and I were and never had a problem with it. I think that part of the reason for that was because I realized, very early on, that he was a far better partner than I was for her, but that I also filled a role in her life that he didn't.

And so, with that as a backdrop, several weeks after she was diagnosed, and just as she was beginning her treatment, I started sending one email to Carla every night, talking about hope and inspiration and seeing beyond the moment and trying to help her get through the night, or to give her something to look forward to in the morning. Over time, a lot of words piled up.

This is not a how-to manual for how to talk to a friend who has cancer or how to be a patient. This is two friends having a (mostly one-sided) conversation - the number of times that she was too sick to even send a text message is too numerous to count. This is one person using his gifts for as much good as he could wring out of them to try to inspire and lift the spirits of their best friend.

This is how it happened, and it is straight from the heart. There are gaps in the chronology, usually because there were days where nothing substantial was happening, but also because this is the nature of dealing with serious illness. Sometimes you don't know everything. So you do the best that you can.

If there is anything that I've learned throughout this time, it is that when your best friend is facing the fight of her life, you do everything you can to tilt the odds in her favor. It is open, honest, ridiculously profane (if you have a problem with the F word and many of its variants, you may find large sections of this uncomfortable), and it was the best way I could express to my friend how much I love her.

Like I said, this isn't a manual or a how-to book. This is what I did. If you have a friend or a close relative facing one of these fights, you need to decide, early on, how much you are willing to do to, how much you are willing to commit to their success. If you're in, you need to be in all of the way. You need to give them all of your energy, all

21

of your faith and hope and belief. Above all, it needs to be unconditional. When they call for help, be there.

Carla and I developed a kind of shorthand over the years. One of our favorite stories was Richard Dreyfuss talking about what it takes to be an actor. His response was surprisingly zen-like: "Look, if you want to be an actor, then you have to BE an actor." I don't want to belabor the point - commit to the task and don't stop.

A couple of logistical notes before we begin:

- The emails will fill in most of the story, but in cases where further explanation of the narrative is required, I've tried to do that. These sections will be in italics above the letter from that day to mark them apart from the emails.

- There were also a large number of emails with status updates that I sent out to friends and family over the months of this saga. I've included them as well because they help to advance the story and provide some background, and also because I think they show in some way how this experience changed not just Carla, but me as well. The emails to Carla were about keeping her inspired and focused, not on rehashing that day's medical news, and the emails to family and friends were about me leaning on my support team so that I could better support her.

- I've taken some screen shots of text message conversations that Carla and I had along the way, because in a lot of cases her words advance the story and add to an understanding better than mine do. For those not familiar with the iPhone text message format, the person who you are talking to is named at the top of the screen, my messages to that person are on the right, and their messages to me are on the left.

- The majority of the text messages are not screenshots, because I wanted to make the text searchable in electronic format. I've tried to a) weave them in to the rest of the story as well as I could and b) use them to help advance the story. There are a fair number of them that are joined in the middle of things, without exposition or explanation. I've tried to limit them, but not knowing every single thing is part of the story. Embrace ambiguity.

- As with any relationship, there are a lot of backstories and inside jokes that are not immediately apparent to someone who is not privy to our history. I was going to use asterisks to manage and explain these things, but I hate asterisks, so you'll find explanations of the references as italicized parentheticals at the end of each day's entry where appropriate.

- In some cases, people and situations and characters will pop in and out and never be fully explained. I was driving myself crazy during the editing process trying to figure out how to explain these things in a way that did not disrupt the narrative. Without giving too much away, I found myself in at the Ryoan-ji Buddhist temple, located in the hills above Kyoto, this past year, and saw their 600-year old rock garden. The 15 stones are placed, it is said, so that no matter where you sit, you are unable to see all of the rocks. The point is that you never know or see all, and so it is with some of the side stories and characters that drop in and out here.

- One of the things that Carla and I share is a love of movies and pop culture. Actually, an unhealthy love of pop culture. There have been numerous instances of us having entire conversations just by using movie references, and so, when writing to her, I often would make a movie reference and then talk about how it applied to whatever was happening at the time. There are so many things in pop culture, while undeniably cheesy, that do carry the ring of truth to them, and given our relationship, and the way that she and I communicate, it was easy to use them as I wrote to her in an attempt to inspire and to motivate her. I've used notes at the end of each day's letter where appropriate to designate these passages.

- The origin of our use of movie references to communicate is lost to the mists of time, but probably traces most of its history to a line from High Fidelity, a film from 2000 starring John Cusack: "...I agreed that what really matters is what you like, not what you are like... Books, records, films - these things matter." These things matter to both of us, and because they do, they had a higher meaning for us both, plus it allowed us to communicate in ways that went beyond just the letters on the page. Then again, her favorite bad movie is "Road House" and mine is "Armageddon". I never claimed that we had great taste.

- There is one exception to the endnotes approach, because quite frankly I got tired of writing the same one again and again. I use the phrase "Adapt. Improvise. Overcome." about a zillion times. It comes from one of my favorite underrated movies, Heartbreak Ridge, which came out in 1986 and starred Clint Eastwood. The phrase is an absolute perfect summary of the things that Carla needed to do to survive and to thrive.

- I've included, amongst the emails, roughly 120 or so text messages that Carla and I exchanged during this time period. Some will note, despite my nearly insane level of hate for typos, that there are a lot of them in her messages. This was on purpose – I copied what she said exactly in order to show the toll that her fight took on her. She was often so tired, or so afflicted by "chemo brain", that this was the best she could do. I include the typos to honor just how much effort was involved in even sending what she did.

Finally, Carla did not just have Stu and I and close family and friends to help her. The cast of individuals helping her out seemed to grow on a daily basis. There are, however, a couple of characters in this story that need some explanation.

- The Naturopath: He is a naturopath / acupuncturist in Seattle that I met through an ex-girlfriend, and who I had personal experience with. As the ex-girlfriend who introduced us says, "he is very simply a Healer." She's right. His whole-patient approach to medicine is something that the medical industry could learn quite a bit from, and he was essential in keeping Carla's spirit nourished at the same time as he was aiding in her medical treatment plan. Carla literally could not have done what she did without his help. I'm not identifying him because getting an appointment with him is already difficult enough.

- The Fox: my father, David Sypolt, who died in late 2000. Fox may be gone, but many of the lessons that he drilled into his children have lived on throughout the years, and have become known colloquially as Foxisms within our circles of friends. Foxisms pepper my conversations with Carla for the same reason that the movie references do - because they are an excellent way to make a point, and you don't need to be a Zen master to grasp their impact.

Even after writing, reading, re-reading, editing and revising this story about a bazillion times, I'm still not sure how to classify it. At its heart, it is the story of a year in my best friend's life, and I am deeply honored to be able to tell it. Or, if you're British, I'm deeply honoured. But my problem with superfluous "u's" is best left for another time, in another story.

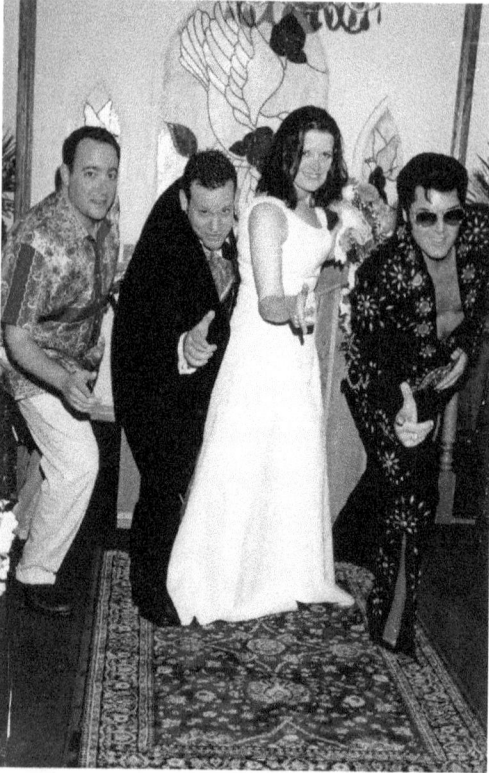

Myself, Stu, Carla, and Elvis during much happier times. At their wedding in May 2003.

January

(Carla and I made her first visit to The Naturopath. She walked out just saying "wow" for about ten minutes).

Text Messages: 1/24/12 7:54 PM

Carla: Can't thank you enough. I am feeling so much better, physically and emotionally.

Me: Thank The Naturopath. He's really just amazing. Wait until he gets his hands on you. I'm really happy that he is able to provide you with help and hope.

Me: We're going to put all of the tools in place for you to win this one, and I think he's going to be a valuable piece of the puzzle.

Carla: Sorry to be so short. Bad night tonight.

1/29/12 - Day One

(After the initial diagnosis, there was a time period of a couple of weeks where not a whole lot was going on. There were tests for Carla to undergo, and a treatment plan to map out, and a whole lot of waiting and worrying. Finally, the time for the first phase of her treatment was at hand - 6 weeks of daily radiation and chemotherapy.)

You can do this. It won't be easy, but you can do this. You have it in you to overcome it. I've seen it in you.

I'm thinking specifically of a moment in 1999 where you were completely freaked out about delivering a speech to more than 6 people. Not even close as far as seriousness is concerned. At the same time, you've conquered a lot of things.

You've overcome scary things in the past. You can do it again. As you said, this will likely be the most difficult thing you've ever done. But you can do it. I remember specifically something you told me recently - that the thing you admire about me is that I am willing to go off in a different direction regardless of what anyone thought.

You can do this. You will do this. You are strong enough to do it, and when it seems too much, you have a large number of people who want to help you. Call on them. Call on me, and Stu, and your friends, and your sister. You have to do this by yourself, but you're not doing it alone.

Here's something I was thinking about recently:

"Is too far!"

No, is not too far. Is just far enough, and you can do this.

I am amongst a large number of people who love and support you. Today is day one. The number of days you have to endure is shrinking.

Is not too far. You can do this. Call me when you think you can't. I love you, and there's a long list of people who want to say the same thing.

(On the subject of "Is Too Far!" - When Carla and Stu eloped to Vegas, I went with them, mainly because I wanted to go to Vegas. The wedding was just the cherry on top. We took a car service to the airport, and the driver mistakenly dropped us off at the opposite end of the terminal from where we needed to be. He realized his mistake after we had started down into the airport and offered to drive us down to the far end. We were ok with walking, but the last thing we heard the driver yelling out was "Is too far!" These inside stories are not going to be all that insightful.)

1/30/12 - Random Thoughts Of The Day

You said that you liked getting the e-mail today, so I think what I'm going to do as part of my contribution to you getting better is to try to write something every night so you have something to look forward to every morning.

Actually, writing is something that I've been doing an awful lot of lately. It seems like when a crisis of some kind comes along in my life, my normally excessive output multiplies. I've already started pre-writing the trip report for TripAdvisor. Days one and two come in at just over 2,000 words, and I haven't even described my activities yet. It took me 15 paragraphs to even get to the part where I was boarding the plane. The legend of SeattleRoyHobbs will either grow beyond measure or I'm going to bore the living crap out of a lot of people. As you said when I got into it with the Seattle Times writer - "those poor dumb bastards."

I went to see The Naturopath today, mainly to ask him what I needed to do to help, to get my mind right (I'm bouncing back and forth between denial and denial and, in my finer moments, super-denial) and to get a feel for what you will be experiencing. He was really positive (without discussing specifics of your case), and he talked a lot about the fact that the main thing that will happen is that you're going to be pretty tired, and that the pain you've experienced will diminish. He also stressed that your medical team will be checking you on a daily basis.

Before I went in, I had a chance to scan one of the books in his office - this one was about a natural way to fight cancer. While I think that a lot of this stuff is unproven, one thing jumped out to me - in 1900 or so, the nationwide cancer rate was 1 in 33 adults. Now it is approaching 1 in 3. There has to be a link to the toxins that are all around us.

That's why I thought that the fact that you're trying to clear all the toxins from your life while simultaneously pumping new medically-approved ones in sounds pretty retarded if you look at it from that angle. Still, it is the best that science has found so far, and it is the best way to shrink down Herman so that you can become an active part of the attack by actually being able to eat.

Today was day one. This was your line in the sand - from now on, Herman is no longer in control, no longer growing. Today is the first day that Herman worries about his future. Tonight Herman has the 3 am moments while you rest and attack. You're in control now, and nobody is coming to his aid.

Ok, about the Herman part - there was a Magnum PI episode from 1984 where Magnum was knocked off his surfski, and at one point was being circled by a tiger shark. To calm himself, he nicknamed the shark Herman (explained in a flashback scene that was revealed later) and eventually told Herman to go away. Since it was TV, Herman left. At the same time, I've used it as shorthand when something worthy of concern comes into my life. Maybe that helps, maybe it doesn't. Maybe it puts the point on the fact that I've watched too much TV in my life.

But the point is that today was important. You're no longer a victim. You're not even defending any more - you're attacking. Every day your opponent grows weaker. Keep eliminating toxins, keep doing what you can every day to get a little bit stronger and to supplement your immune system, and soon you'll be able to take an even more active role.

I hate ending on sort of a down note, so here's my favorite joke - I may have told it to you in the past, so bear with me:

Friday around 4:30 or so in a research facility. One researcher is walking by another researcher's office. The guy in the office is holding an apple and staring off into space.

"What's the deal with the apple?"

"I have invented an apple that tastes just like pussy."

"Really? Let me try it."

The apple is tossed to the first guy, who takes a bite and immediately spits it out.

"That tastes like shit!"

"Of course it does. Turn it around."

Rest up and prepare for the fight. It may not feel like it, but you are already winning.

(An explanation of the TripAdvisor reference - I was scheduled to take a vacation on Maui from 2/4 until 2/19. I debated about canceling or rescheduling, but Carla was insistent that I go on my trip, as it had been booked since a rainy 43 degree day in May the previous year. Seattle weather can sometimes border on the ridiculous.)

Text Messages: 1/31/12 5:53 PM

Me: I'm going to proceed on the assumption that you're trying to rest, so I won't call unless you tell me it is OK rather than disturbing you.

Carla: I am trying to rest. Another very bad day at the dr. The promise this will be the last one for a while. I'm just trying to lay down until the pain passes.

Me: I figured as much. Herman is having a much worse day than you are, if that helps.

Carla: I fucking hope so! Bastard!

Me: He's all alone in this, and the bartender keeps making him drink like it is the shot contest in Raiders.

Carla: Wow I really hope for as sick as I am right now that this is all working!! This is hard.

Me: I can't even imagine. Can you handle a phone call?

Carla: No. Can't talk. Can barely breathe. Stu is running to group health to get me some meds.

Carla: Did not expect the side effects to kick in this fast.

Me: Just imagine how hard it is on Herman. No friends. No hope. You can get through this. You are loved by so many people. The hard will end soon. You are stronger than this. I know it. I love you more than anything. You can do it.

Carla: Thank you. That helps.

Me: The Naturopath gave me a great exercise for meditation: as you breathe in, say the word "bliss". As you breathe out, say the word "attachment".

Me: So much of our hurt can be traced to becoming attached to something - either some future goal, or to something that happened to us in the past.

Me: Breathe it out. Diminish its power by expelling it via your breath.

Carla: That is actually helping. Thanks.

February

Text Messages: 2/1/12 9:43 PM

Carla: Comes and goes but much less intense than yesterday.

Me: Good. When you want to talk or text, I'm here. Keep breathing in bliss and breathing out attachment.

Carla: Thank you. It really does help. I told friends about Herman and they shared with others so Herman has an entire hit squad after him now.

Me: And not just a regular hit squad. Those people will get medieval on him.

2/1/12 - Really? I'm the Tony Robbins of Cancer?

The news that you're feeling better today than the first 2 days is welcome indeed. Hopefully you've experienced the worst it is going to throw at you - it left you woozy but still standing. That's important to know. Embrace the strength that you displayed. Embrace the fact that you have it within you to keep going. Embrace the fact that you're going to win.

Just as important is that you're napalming the ever-loving crap out of Herman. You have to know that the toll that this took on you over two days is taking an even greater toll on him, and you get to see the effects (hopefully) on Friday when they run the tests on you.

You have the distinction of being the first person I've ever known who has cancer. Congratulations on taking my cherry - one more thing that you have going for you.

Since you're my first, I've been at a loss to try to figure out how I can help. I found a local support group for friends and family that I start going to after I get back from Maui. I'm not looking to share feelings, etc. (most people know, of course, that I don't share or play well with others) but I'm more looking for ideas about how I and the rest of Team Carla can help support you. I think it comes down to making things as easy as possible on you. As I learn stuff, I'll pass it along to you or the rest of the team.

I don't want to dwell on last night, as I have learned my lesson. I apologize to you and Stu for any anxiety / whatever that I caused by my actions. It shouldn't have happened last night, and it won't happen again.

In the weird things department, you now have a random stranger in Seattle wearing one of your bracelets. A woman in a bar spotted mine and asked what it was for.

She asked me if I had extras, and I did, so somebody that you will likely never meet, and I will never see again, is pulling for you. This is like really primitive social networking. Talking to people – it's the new Facebook!

One question that I do need some direction on - do you want to take over the scheduling of appointments with The Naturopath or do you want me to continue? Given that your other appointment is later in the day, and the 4 pm appointments tend to go pretty quickly according to the receptionist that I talked to, booking as far into the future as possible is advised. They have a 24 hour cancellation policy, so you can wait until the last minute. Better to have the appointment available.

Either way, please let me know, and also please let me know how often you want to go. As you know, I'm the last person you would expect to go in for this stuff, but I've become a True Believer in this guy - the feeling of relief I received on Monday was palpable, and I'd encourage you to take advantage of it as often as you can.

It is early, but starting to plan for life after treatment is something that you might want to think about. Don't spend a lot of time on it, as you need to concentrate on getting better, but try to spend some time deciding who you want to be when you emerge from this.

We touched on it a little bit this weekend, and I think you're in tune with it based on a lot of things that you said. The Naturopath hits me with it pretty much every time I see him. He keeps asking the same question, with almost no variation - what is the story of your life?

When this is behind you, and it will be, sooner than you think, the whole world will lay in front of you. There will be nothing you cannot do. You will have already literally fought for your life, and you will have won. There will be no challenge that you cannot take on.

So if you have a chance, start to think about really being one of the Crazy Ones. The ones who think different. Because the people who are crazy enough to think that they can change the world are the ones who do. You're one of those people. You've known it for a long time. Take this time to rest and prepare and plot and plan to take your passion to the next level.

Have a great day and I look forward to hearing from you soon.

Text Messages: 2/2/12 6:29 PM

Me: How did it go this afternoon?

Carla: It goes okay but the pain afterwards is terrible, I had to take a valium in order to calm down and stop crying. Fuck fuck fuck this better be working.

Me: It is working. Herman is getting his ass kicked. You can do this. You're tougher than anyone I know.

Carla: I'm afraid I'm all bark and no bite!!

Me: No. You've got plenty of bite. I've been on the receiving end enough times to verify that fact.

Carla: Well I just wish I'd had a few fistfights in my life. Then I would feel truly badass.

Me: We can arrange for that after your treatment is done.

Carla: Maybe that is the them of my remission party. Fight Club!

Me: We don't talk about Fight Club. You should know better than that. We'll just invite people who have pissed you off in the past and you can take your best shots.

Carla: If I start punching guests at the onset of the party I am thinking we would clear the place pretty fast.

2/2/12 - Tonight's Update

It sounds like today was difficult. I'm sorry to hear that. Everything that I've read tells me that the early parts are the hardest, and that it does get easier from a physical standpoint. The sooner that you can start eating, the better.

You are winning. Herman keeps having a succession of bad days. You're going to win this one.

You're only 7 days away from your first time where The Naturopath gets to do stuff to you. Do you remember how you felt after just talking to him? Wait until he gets his hands on you. You know me - I wouldn't be saying these things unless I Believed with a capital B.

I don't want to oversell this, but I ask you to trust me that he's a transformative figure. I can't describe it - you have to experience it for yourself.

One small piece of advice, at least for the first couple of sessions - don't include whoever drove you. While I was grateful to be able to be there, you can unlock stuff one-on-one that you can't unlock if someone else is in the room.

As Morpheus said after Neo visits the Oracle in The Matrix: "what is said there is for you, and you alone." I don't think I need to spell out how this applies to you.

In other completely unrelated news, it looks like we are moving our offices to a building on Dexter. I suspect that many of us will have transition problems as we move in - this space is awesome, including an amazing water view of South Lake Union. Moving out of our crappy offices is going to be a huge step up.

It is difficult to imagine that the little company with a shack in the backyard filled with metal has grown up. I look at the numbers every day and can't even comprehend them.

Let's get back to the important stuff: Carla - you've gotten through things that I cannot even imagine. You're stronger than this, and you've demonstrated an ability to adapt and overcome. You are the Big C. Herman is your bitch. Maybe not today, but soon.

It will happen.

In the meantime, you have a random chick that none of us will ever see wearing your bracelet. Which is nice.

You can do this. You've already done the hard part. Herman is on the ropes - finish him. Take him out to the woodshed and make him your bitch. Imagine that he is Ned Beatty in Deliverance.

He's dead, whether he knows it or not. You're going to kick his ass, no matter what it takes. You've already demonstrated that.

Never give up. Never surrender. You're the best that I've ever met, and you can do this.

Text Messages: 2/3/12 12:38 PM

Carla: Me too and I hope that it lasts. Thanks for last nights entry I loved it.

Me: Glad to hear that you are enjoying them and that they are helping in some small way.

Carla: They help in a BIG way. They are my daily affirmation and motivation. I read and re-read them everyday.

Me: You're going to give me a swelled head. Just trying to give you as much support as I possibly can.

Carla: Well it's working.

2/3/12 - You're nothing less than awesome

Loved hearing my best friend's voice tonight, and the optimism that you had. You're going to win.

I knew something wasn't right this week. I can't really describe how good it felt to hear the happiness in your voice tonight. I am so happy for you that they've figured out the things that work for you.

You've survived the worst that they can put you through, and you ate Italian to celebrate, which on Monday was probably the last thing you thought you would be doing.

As it turns out, you're way tougher than you knew you were. It was such a pleasure to hear the optimism in your voice tonight. As we were talking, I knew that this was the time that you had beaten it, although the final score is yet to be determined. Herman has been cut.

From Rocky IV:

"He's cut! He's cut! The Russian is cut!"

(later)

Duke (Rocky's trainer); "You cut him. He's not a machine. He's a man.

Drago: "He's not human. He is like a piece of iron."

You are a piece of iron. They've thrown the worst at you. You are a piece of iron. You will win.

Every time the garbage compactor does its thing, realize that Herman is having a very bad time, and that there is no way out of the garbage chute for him.

Cannot possibly describe how happy I am for you. You're winning, and Herman is now crawling into the fetal position. Finish him. Today was your Independence Day, when you turned the corner.

I quote the President in Independence Day. You're not going to go quietly into the night.

"Good morning. In less than an hour, aircraft from here will join others from around the world. And you will be launching the largest aerial battle in the history of mankind. 'Mankind.' That word should have new meaning for all of us today. We can't be consumed by our petty differences anymore. We will be united in our common interests. Perhaps it's fate that today is the Fourth of July, and you will once again be fighting for our freedom... Not from tyranny, oppression, or persecution... but from annihilation. We are fighting for our right to live. To exist. And should we win the day, the Fourth of July will no longer be known as an American holiday, but as the day the world declared in one voice: 'We will not go quietly into the night! We will not vanish without a fight! We're going to live on! We're going to survive! Today we celebrate our Independence Day!'"

You're already winning. More than that, Herman's time is through.

Easily one of my favorite scenes:

http://www.youtube.com/watch?v=vwpTj_Z9v-c

Now go out there and take it. You've earned this.

(Carla and I did some visualization of Herman, and the best we could come up with was the creature in the garbage compactor in Star Wars, hence the garbage chute stuff above.)

46

2/4/12 - Keeping up the skeer

Wow. Really hard to write these things when you've been drinking for more than 4 hours straight. Where to start?

How about the fact that I woke up with a grin on my face this morning that was a thousand miles wide? Hearing the life in your voice made my day, my week, my month. We haven't talked today, but I hope that it has continued.

I'm actually really looking forward to getting back and meeting the members of your medical team, as well as to talk to the people who have the same appointment time as you. They sound really great.

I love the fact that you went with Italian as your first really solid food. Fuck Herman. He is barely even on your radar any more. Put one of ours on the oncology ward? We'll put three of yours in the morgue. You really were built for this, the more that I think about it.

Civil War history stuff (yes, I do occasionally veer outside of the Pacific War) - General Nathan Bedford Forrest is widely credited with inventing the principle of Deep Strike - hitting an enemy far in his rear and sowing confusion among the typically second-rate soldiers that were found far in the rear.

His second contribution is lesser-known but equally as valuable in your case. He called it "keeping up the skeer" (scare in non-southern English). His principle, as explained by Tom Clancy in Executive Orders, was that once you had your enemy on the run, keep attacking him, keep nipping at his heels. Force him into mistakes.

Even when it really doesn't matter any more.

That's the key - only one of you can exist. It is either you or Herman. So punish him. Don't let up. Accept nothing less than full capitulation. You've got him running. He is hurting. He has nowhere to turn. Don't give him one. Finish him. He's hurt you - return the fucking favor. No fucking mercy.

Keep up the skeer.

(Yes, I am aware that Forrest founded the KKK, but this wasn't a treatise on stupid things that people have done with their lives).

2/5/12 - The Best There Ever Was

Was reading the paper this morning and happened to see this in the horoscope section:

"Persistence in the face of failure is often the key to eventual success, except in skydiving."

You're not skydiving.

That just really jumped out at me. Your first week was not the resounding success that we all hoped it to be. Easy for me to say - you had to actually go through it. I can't tell you how much I Admire (yes, with a capital A - you've earned it) the strength that you've shown in the face of adversity. Now that you know how deep those reserves go, now that you've tapped into them, there is nothing that can stop you. Embrace that.

I assume that you've seen The Natural. There are an insane number of things that you can take away from that movie, but let's look at one thing:

Harriet Byrd: What do you want, Roy?

Roy Hobbs: I want to walk down the street and have people say 'There goes Roy Hobbs, the best there ever was in the game.'

Harriet Byrd: And what about after that?

Roy Hobbs: What else is there?

Once you've killed Herman, you have nothing else to prove. There is nothing else.

You'll walk down the street, and people will say, 'There goes Carla, who killed Herman'. (Supposing, of course, that they've been privy to this long string of emails, and understand who Herman is, and actually recognize you. I'm stretching the boundaries a little - go with me on this.) At any rate, you will have nothing left to prove to anybody.

You're going to walk away from this - you'll be changed, surely. But in the end, nobody can ever take this away from you. You will have shown who you are.

Never surrender. Be the best that there ever was, regardless of whether or not people recognize you on the street.

Text Messages: 2/6/12 6:49 PM

Me: I'm so happy that you've been able to weather the initial storm. You're getting better every day.

Carla: I believe that. I feel that.

Me: And you are laying waste to Herman.

Carla: Every second of everyday.

Me: No mercy. No conditional surrender. This is basically World War II inside your lower intestinal tract, and Herman is the Japanese Empire.

Carla: And I am Unbreakable!

2/7/12 - Let's talk about little t try and Big T Try

Time to revisit something from my distant past. (This is slightly more effective if you play A Little Respect by Erasure as you read it - multimedia inspiration!)

I'm going to spend some time talking about my career path. Eventually it will circle back to you and how this helps. Bear with me. We will get there eventually.

In 1994, once I had decided to leave Continental Aluminum (having decided that dirt in my coffee every day was a bad idea) I had a wide range of options - I was a buyer, and that translates well to any number of industries. Even back then, I was an insanely good resume writer and got a call from Copper & Brass Sales (later purchased by ThyssenKrupp, for those of you keeping score at home).

Of course, because my ex-wife was insanely jealous, I got a phone call at 10 am on a Tuesday:

Her: "Who is Michelle?"

Me: "I have no idea. What are you talking about?"

Her: "I got a call today from somebody named Michelle who wanted to talk to you, but she didn't say what it was about."

(Three days pass)

Her: "That Michelle woman called back and left a message. She works for a company named Copper & Brass Sales and wants to interview you."

Of note – my ex-wife never apologized for nearly costing me an escape route from Continental. Crazy is as crazy does. I am insanely thankful that I got out of both that marriage and Continental Aluminum.

There is something for you eventually. Allow me to tell the story properly. It is likely the only official record of the full saga.

1994-1998 was an amazing time for me. As much as I curse ThyssenKrupp, the experience at Copper & Brass was formative. It helped that my soon to be ex-wife and I grew increasingly apart.

This was the time of the rise of Microsoft Office, when yet another Seattle-based company was laying waste to their competition. The key, for me at least, was that they had created rudimentary programming tools. All you needed to take advantage of them was time and curiosity.

I have always had an abnormal level of curiosity. My ex-wife provided the time, as she would disappear for days on end, with no explanation where she had been. I could see the end coming, but wasn't willing to admit to it.

At the same time, I was plumbing the depths of Office. I learned something new every day (and/or night), and I would apply it at work.

I was able to finesse a transfer from purchasing to sales. Not the most politically correct move. Still, it had to be done as I'd gotten to the point that I was really bored with Purchasing - it was just the same math again and again. I continued my exploration of Excel and Access.

Eventually, the position of Inside Sales Manager opened up. The candidates for the job were asked to submit a resume and a Plan for 12 Months. It will not surprise you that my plan for 12 months spanned 40 pages. I have never been afflicted with brevity.

Jumping ahead, mainly because the narrative is bogging down, I didn't get that job. I eventually figured out that I had been trying (with a capital T) too hard to get to the next step on the management ladder.

I failed in that attempt. But all of the skills I had discovered over several years of little t trying were exactly what I needed during the early years at OnlineMetals.

How does this relate to you, I imagine that you are asking after about 20 paragraphs.

Your fight with Herman isn't a single battle - it happens every day. It isn't Big T Try. It is little t try. Every single day. In my case, it was learning something new. In your case, it is being strong enough to take out more of Herman.

I can't really express how much I admire your resilience, your patience, and your strength. You are winning. Soon you will have a lot of extra help.

And then you'll put a bullet in Herman's brain.

Focus on the little things that you are doing to hasten his demise. Denying him milk and all of its life-giving proteins and hormones. Oh, and the 24-hour supply of poison. Basically, the worst parts of Iocaine Powder.

You're killing him. It isn't easy. But you're going to do it. Money never sleeps? You know what else doesn't sleep? Chemo targeted at Herman. He's dead. He just doesn't know it yet.

You're going to beat him. Keep up the skeer, keep up your strength, keep attacking, no matter how you feel. No mercy. You have a deep support team to help you. Lean on us when you waver, but don't ever stop the assault.

You're going to break him, as long as you keep doing the things required by little t try.

I love you and support you. If you need anything, call.

Have a great day.

Text Messages: 2/7/12 7:15 PM

Me: How goes it this evening? I wish I could report to you that I was looking at a beautiful sunset, but the truth is that it is raining cats and dogs. Actually more cats than dogs, but that is splitting hairs.

Carla: Well I wish I had something good to report but the last two days have been grueling. The side effects have been especially brutal today. A lot of deep breathing and tears.

Me: You're going to do this. Herman keeps weakening. I truly believe that at the end there will be no need for surgery, as he can't stand up to the fire hose of poison that your team is directing at him.

Carla: I believe that too. He is being obliterated every minute of every day.

2/8/12 - Your own personal Seal Team Six

Once you get better, even if I have to strap you down and read it to you, Cryptonomicon by Neal Stephenson is in your future.

One line sticks out for me - "On Guadalcanal, the Americans and Japanese are contesting, with rifles, their right to build an airfield."

I've read an awful lot about Guadalcanal - if not for the courage of about ten thousand Marines, who decided that this was a line that the Japanese could not be allowed to cross, the war would have ended differently. Those Marines easily would have recognized you as one of their own.

It also helped that the Japanese had only one approach to battle, and it was one that had a giant weakness.

Your enemy is not that different - while it seems to be everywhere, it does have a weakness, in that its cells divide quickly. Your team is attacking that vulnerability. As an aside, why does it seem that every evil influence seems to leave one glaring weakness?

Your team is winning. Every single day. Trust them. They are your own personal Seal Team Six. It doesn't feel like it, but Herman is a Dead Man Walking. He's up for execution, and the governor is out of town.

For God and Country. Geronimo, Geronimo, EKIA.

Herman is on the list. He only thinks that he is safe. That will end soon.

Carla. Fuck Yeah.

2/9/12 - The Wheels on the Bus

I remember, very distinctly, during my second Seattle Super Skate from Redmond to Seattle, having gotten about halfway through, when everything seemed to be against me. My legs felt dead. The terrain was uphill. The wind was coming at me.

"Please, Fox," I remember saying. "A little help would be nice."

The wind shifted directions soon after that, and you and I, as well as my insanely large calves, went out for brunch.

For the longest time, I denied the existence of a higher power, but the older that I get, and the more that I see, the more I want to believe.

The thing that got me through the early years at OnlineMetals (OLM) was simple - I refused to accept defeat, and I knew I was right at a level that is hard to explain. I knew that the basic business had legs, if only we could keep it alive. John wanted to shut it down 3 or 4 times, but I refused to yield.

So let's start with the basics - fix it in your mind that you refuse to accept defeat. It is not an option. No retreat. No surrender. Ever.

And if you need to ask for a little tailwind, I believe that Fox is there to provide it.

Finally - I'll explain the circumstances when I get back, but I met Jerome Bettis today - the man who I am still convinced tried to kill me with a goal-line fumble in 2006 during the Steelers-Colts Divisional Round playoff game, and will be in the Hall of Fame soon.

Can't wait to tell you the story. I love you and know that you're stronger than Herman. You will outplay, outlast, and outwit him.

Keep fighting. You are invincible.

(Fox is my family's nickname for my dad, David Sypolt, who passed a lot of wisdom on to his kids. Or, actually, anybody who would listen. You will hear from him again. And again. And again.)

Text Messages: 2/10/12 9:37 AM

Me: Ok. Hang in there. You're stronger than Herman and I'm so proud of you for how much you've accomplished so far. Be invincible, no matter how much it feels like you aren't.

2/10/12 - Don't accept mediocrity

One of the overriding themes from the Steve Jobs book is that accepting Mediocrity is basically accepting failure.

Do not accept mediocrity. You're killing Herman, every single day. Soon he will have no power over you.

You can get through this. You are 1/3 of the way there. Before you know it, you will be 2/3 of the way. You're stronger than he is. You have a far deeper support system.

You're going to win. Keep doing what you're doing. He has no chance to survive. Don't let up. Don't give a moment to breathe. Keep pushing.

As I've said before, the Big C is Carla. This is your house. As Matt Damon says in Dogma, Who's house? Carla's house! Nobody comes in to your house and pushes you around.

Be Invincible. He can hurt you, but he cannot wound you. You're too strong for that.

2/11/12 - The Gutsiest Move I Ever Saw

One of my proudest moments was the night I won over $5,000 on Blackjack at the Flamingo 4 or 5 years ago.

Fox started showing me the rules of blackjack when I was probably 6 years old. By the time I visited Vegas the first time, I knew the rules backwards and forwards, and yet, in my first time in a live game, I froze.

The dealer had a 5 showing, and I asked for another card. The look on the face of The Fox was akin to sheer horror. What had he raised? How had he failed in this way?

I recovered after a moment and made the correct play. Over the years, I developed a deep understanding for the math behind the game, which is as beautiful as it is frustrating.

And so I found myself, 6 or 7 years later, playing blackjack at the Flamingo. I started out playing $25 a hand, which was expensive but doable. Fox had taught me that once you were playing with house money, it was imperative that you keep betting at high levels - that was the only way that you could keep ahead. His rules said that when you win, you increase your bet.

On this night, I had won enough that I went from $25/hand to $600/hand. I had won over $6,000 in about an hour. This is when the 8's came.

Anytime you're playing blackjack, and you see a pair of 8's, the rule is to always split them. Against a dealer 10, they are worthless. Against a dealer showing 6, they are a weapon. This dealer was showing a 6.

I split the 8's, and two more 8's came out. Two more 8's. Then a pair of 3's on top of the 8's. I doubled my bet on the eights and threes, and all of a sudden I had 6 hands going at the same time.

At $600/hand, plus $100 per hand for the dealers.

The dealer pulled the face-down card, which was a 10, giving her 16, then pulled another 10, which broke her.

In the revelry that followed, I remember only one thing - one of the younger pit bosses came up to me and said "everyone plays that wrong - gutsiest move I've ever seen, Maverick." That's a line straight out of Top Gun, and I had to give the 23 year old who uttered it credit.

What's the lesson here? You're splitting 8's and doubling down on 11. All, and I do mean all, of the odds are in your favor. You just have to have the guts to make it work for you.

Herman is dying. Stay the course. You can do this. You can sit at this table.

Gutsiest move I ever saw? Hah! You've displayed the gutsiest move I've ever seen. Don't let up. Don't surrender. Keep up the skeer. Chase him down, even when it doesn't matter any more.

Text Messages: 2/12/12 6:19 PM

Carla: Up and down. Riding the tide.

Me: 1/3 of this is behind you. You're winning. Keep it in your head and your heart that this is hurting him way more than it is you. You're going to be free of him soon.

Carla: I hope so. This past week was very tought.

Me: And you were tougher.

2/12/12 - The Life You Learn With

Let's go back to The Natural for a moment -

Iris Gaines: You know, I believe we have two lives.

Roy Hobbs: How...what do you mean?

Iris Gaines: The life we learn with and the life we live with after that.

You're going to live two distinctive lives. As The Naturopath said, this is the curse and the gift of cancer.

I think I've talked in the past about his obsession with asking one very simple question: "what is the story of your life?" He's asked me that no less than a dozen times, so I'm making an assumption that he thinks it is important. (I have a pet theory about him, but that is for a different time.)

At the same time, trying to connect the dots from your past to your future is nearly impossible. I look back at the things that made me, and there's no way that 20-year-old me, or 30-year-old me, or even 40-year-old me would have ever seen what I have become.

The point is that everything that you've learned along the way, and everything that you're experiencing now, is laying the foundation for everything that you're going to become. You just have no idea which puzzle pieces are most important.

You're 1/3 of the way through. You've taken Herman's best shot. He keeps getting weaker, and you're getting stronger, no matter how you feel at the moment. You're winning. We both know this.

Start planning for your future. Start planning to connect the dots of your past into the story of the rest of your life. Become who you were meant to be, but have always held back from because of what others might think.

Do not waste this gift, even though right now it feels like a curse. You're stronger than anyone I know, and you're going to win.

After that, you're going to change the world. I have no idea how, but I've seen it in you. All you have to do in order to step through that door is to believe that you can. The first step is believing that you're going to win. After that, every step will be both easy and clear.

I love you and believe in you. You are unstoppable. Keep powering through.

2/13/12 - Lessons From The Spoon Boy

Spoon boy: "Do not try and bend the spoon. That's impossible. Instead... only try to realize the truth."

Neo: "What truth?"

Spoon boy: "There is no spoon."

Neo: "There is no spoon?"

Spoon boy: "Then you'll see, that it is not the spoon that bends, it is only yourself."

Oh yes, we are going there. This may feel like a physical battle, and down in your bowels, a war is raging. But more than anything, this is a mental war. You need to decide, here and now, that you're going to prevail. You're Invincible. You're Unbreakable. Be those things.

In the early days of World War II, Admiral Yamamoto wrote a letter in which he predicted that if Japan went to war, in the first 6 months he would run wild, but after that, the industrial might of the US would destroy Japan.

Admiral William "Bull" Halsey had a different spin on things:

"When this war is over," he said, "Japanese will be spoken only in Hell."

Not sure that you know the rest of the story - American code breakers deciphered a set of messages detailing Yamamoto's itinerary on a morale-building tour. His plane was intercepted, at extreme range, by 8 P-38's over Bougainville Island in 1943.

Your medical team is just as ruthless. Trust them to do their job and to cut off all of Herman's hope of escape.

Don't let up. Herman is in his death throes - the only way to be sure of it is to keep doing what you're doing. Make sure that his language is spoken only in Hell.

Morpheus: "What are you waiting for? You're faster than this. Don't think you are, know you are. Come on. Stop trying to hit me and hit me."

Don't try to hit him. Hit him. Again and again.

Enjoy your time with The Naturopath and have a great day. I love you and I Believe in you. Keep winning.

2/14/12 - Something Larger

I'll confess that I have a little bit of writer's block tonight - I can write, but after the output of the last week or so, including the notes I've taken for future TripAdvisor posts, I don't have a whole lot of new stuff.

I'm glad to hear that you and The Naturopath are connecting, and that you're able to tap into his reservoir. While our conversation today wasn't that deep, I could hear in your voice that he is providing some reassurance in your fight.

More than that, he's tapping into something that you realized a long time ago - there is something more, something that can't be touched by the physical. It isn't fair that you've had to go through this to reveal it, but it is there with you, every single day.

The obvious cliche is the Footsteps poster (God: the single set of footsteps was when I carried you, yada, yada, yada). I personally don't know if I agree with that, but listening to you, hearing your voice, and reading your texts, I've opened up to the fact that there is something beyond the physical realm that keeps us moving forward. You've gotten through 2-1/2 weeks of a grueling regimen (more like 6-1/2 weeks if you consider how long you waited between diagnosis and treatment - hey - you're in the home stretch!)

How did you do that? How did you get through it? What kept you going at 3 AM? There are two possible answers that I can come up with: one is your own personal resolve that you are not going to let something named Herman beat you. Seriously - Herman? Who the hell is named Herman in the last 50 years? The other answer is that you've tapped into something larger, something that we can't prove exists. Something that can help you power through.

Roy Hobbs: Why did you stand up?

Iris Gaines: Because I didn't want to see you fail.

I am the last person that you would ever expect to be delivering this message, but I am coming to find the truth in it - there is a larger force that we are dimly aware of, and that shows its face from time to time.

I finished Unbroken several days ago and was horrified, rather than inspired. It made me angry that The Bird got away. But all of the men that Louie encountered should have been dead by the end of the story - there is no way any of them should have been able to withstand the physical attacks and the deprivation of food and dignity for 2+ years.

They tapped into something else.

Ray Kinsella: "You once wrote, 'every so often the cosmic tumblers click into place, and the universe opens up, and shows you what's possible'"

Tap into it, whatever it is. It can help you get through the times when you think it is too far.

It is never, ever too far. You've proven that you can do this. Keep pushing. You're almost through. Herman looks bad and feels worse.

I love you and Believe in you.

Text Messages: 2/15/12 6:54 PM

Me: Checking in and hope that you had a good day. Keep winning, keep fighting, keep kicking Herman's ass. Believe it - you're doing it, and I couldn't be prouder of you.

Carla: Thank you coach. You definitely keep me going!!

2/15/12 - Not sure of a subject. Let's go with "A Journey"

[Luke can't levitate his X-Wing out of the bog]

Luke: I can't. It's too big.

Yoda: Size matters not. Look at me. Judge me by my size, do you? Hmm? Hmm. And well you should not. For my ally is the Force, and a powerful ally it is. Life creates it, makes it grow. Its energy surrounds us and binds us. Luminous beings are we, not this crude matter. You must feel the Force around you; here, between you, me, the tree, the rock, everywhere, yes. Even between the land and the ship.

[Using the Force, Yoda effortlessly frees the X-Wing from the bog]

Luke: I don't, I don't believe it.

Yoda: That is why you fail.

(Empire Strikes Back, from the good Trilogy).

Luminous beings we are, beyond this crude matter. As much as I want to napalm George Lucas for episodes I-III, he gave us a great insight. Do not stop believing.

I cannot believe I'm pasting the following. Then again, I am not above cheating. I draw the line, however, at

searching YouTube for the video. There are some things
that are beyond the pale.
(More stuff after the lyrics)

Just a small town girl, livin' in a lonely world
She took the midnight train goin' anywhere
Just a city boy, born and raised in south Detroit
He took the midnight train goin' anywhere

A singer in a smoky room
A smell of wine and cheap perfume
For a smile they can share the night
It goes on and on and on and on

(Chorus)
Strangers waiting, up and down the boulevard
Their shadows searching in the night
Streetlights people, living just to find emotion
Hiding, somewhere in the night.

Working hard to get my fill,
Everybody wants a thrill
Payin' anything to roll the dice,
Just one more time
Some will win, some will lose
Some were born to sing the blues
Oh, the movie never ends
It goes on and on and on and on

(Chorus)

Don't stop believin'
Hold on to the feelin'
Streetlights people

Don't stop believin'
Hold on
Streetlight people

Don't stop believin'
Hold on to the feelin'
Streetlights people

Be well and have a great day kicking Herman's ass. Size matters not - engage your luminous self.

I love you and (yes, I am about to say this) DON'T STOP BELIEVING, HOLD ONTO THAT FEELING.

(I freely admit that this was not my finest hour or best writing. Not every thing can be perfect every day.)

Text Messages: 2/16/12 6:29 PM

Me: Checking in - you're almost halfway. Every day is part of a declining number of days to deal with this - celebrate the fact that you're shown your fangs to Herman.

Me: You may not feel like it sometimes, but you've been indomitable. Keep up the pressure on Herman.

Carla: I'm trying and thanks for the words of encouragement. Lots of pain tonight. Just doing my best to breathe through it.

Me: You're not just trying. You're doing.

2/16/12 - Go That Way, Really Fast. When You See Something, Turn

Quite a bit of ground to cover this morning.

Your sister was kind enough to call me and give me an update. I've tried not to call that much because I expect by now that you're tired of answering questions about how you're doing and how you're feeling. I am very much looking forward to talking to you on Monday when I get back. This trip has not necessarily lived up to expectations.

At any rate, she told me how you're doing - that your color is good, you've lost some weight, but that you look great and that you're kicking Herman's ass. I was gratified to hear from her - she is so totally your cheerleader.

One of the things that she told me in a text earlier today triggered something that led to a little bit of research. Basically, at 2 or so your time, she said that you had had a good morning but as the time for the visit to the docs had approached, you were becoming more stressed.

Way back in 1998, when CBS was looking at me for a management position, they subjected me to a battery of standardized tests to see if I was a good fit for them - one of the things that came out was that I'm insanely good at spotting trends - I can feel them before they become obvious.

What I'm seeing here is a trend (mind you, I'm piecing this together from observations and guesses - there is a chance that I'm completely off - but I don't think so.)

The more time that passes after the treatment, the better that things get for you, until sometime in the midmorning, when you start thinking about what is in store for the afternoon, and your anxiety level rises.

This is all absolutely normal. The research I've done shows that the anticipation of a painful experience is in many cases worse than the actual experience. This has been documented in about a dozen studies in the last 5 years.

I can tell you from personal experience that this phenomenon exists - I didn't go to the dentist for a decade and had to go through 3 root canals as a result. The anticipation and the anxiety before the first one was awful - I felt like I was going to crawl out of my skin. By the time of the third one, I was able to deal with the pain, because I had conquered my pre-appointment anxiety.

You can conquer your anxiety.

I'm not saying any of this to minimize what you're feeling - clearly, what happens post-radiation is beyond anything I can imagine, or want to imagine.

But you've done this, and you've proven that you're stronger than everything that has been thrown at you. You have exactly nothing to fear, and by extension, you have nothing to be anxious about. Breathe.

The Naturopath will remind you that there is the past, which you can't do anything about, and there is the future, which you can influence, but presents a danger if you attach too much to one particular outcome. What remains is the Now, which you experience now. And now. And now. And now. And now. And now. And now.

Live and exist in the moment. Do not allow the future to determine your experience now. Do not allow what is going to happen 4 hours from now, or what you believe is going to happen 4 hours from now, to determine how you feel now. And now. And now.

Live in the moment. Enjoy the periods of calm. Remember them when times are difficult. You can get back there. Your natural state is to be calm.

I know that there is a lot of risk in sending you this message right now, but I talked to your sister, and I spent a lot of time thinking about you. I know that if it was me, I would want to realize what was going on, and I would want to hear this. Eventually, I sent your sister an email detailing my thoughts. Her response: "tell her."

As smart as you are, you've probably realized the cycle that is happening. There are some tools that can help:

- Yoga - get your body moving when it feels good. Nothing bad can happen as a result of this.

- Meditation - much the same as yoga, get your head into the right place to continue the fight.

- Weed - it is supposed to be good for anxiety. Try it out before you go, rather than after.

- See The Naturopath before your normal appointment in order to release the anxiety instead of after. He has 3 appointments this upcoming week and a lot the following week. I know from personal experience how amazing he is at releasing anxiety.

OK - now that you have endured and discarded the practical portion of today's program, let's talk about next steps.

Today marks, for you, the halfway point. After the first couple of days, after the first week, you never thought you'd get here.

But here you stand. Stand is an important word. You've taken what they can throw at you, and you're still here. You cannot be knocked down. You cannot be forced to waver. You are a piece of iron. You haven't backed down one inch.

I've finally figured you out - you're part Weeble-Wobble. Kidding. Sort of. Ok, not really kidding.

Decide that you will not accept failure. Herman is a shell of himself. You remain who you have always been. All that is left to do is to send in the body bag, which will happen soon enough.

Believe in what you are doing. Create your world with your breath and your words. Tap in to the life force when you need it - it is there for you. Above all, recognize how much strength you've shown already. Feel your strength radiating outward. You can do this, and the proof is that you already have.

You're the strongest person that I've ever known. After this is over, you have nothing to prove to anybody. After this is over, you're going to be the best motivational speaker on the planet.

Start planning for your future. Start planning to change the world. Start being one of the Crazy Ones.

I love you and I believe in you.

2/16/12 - Email to my Aunt Kazuko

Hi Kaz -

I'm very sorry to have missed you on this trip, but I completely understand why we won't be able to connect this time.

This has been both a good and a difficult trip for me - about a month ago, my best friend Carla was diagnosed with stage 3 colon cancer. She started chemo and radiation, which will last 6 weeks, the week before I left.

I had really mixed emotions about coming, but she told me to come out and to get my mind ready to provide support for her when I got back - she had her husband, sister, and some other friends to lean on while I was away.

Since I can't be there to support her in person, I've taken it upon myself to write her an email every night focusing on inspiration, perseverance, and belief. Looking back, I've written nearly 15,000 words over almost 3 weeks.

I wasn't sure how much of an impact I was making until a text message exchange we had a week or so ago:

Her: "Thanks for last night's entry. I loved it!"

Me: "Glad to hear that you are enjoying them and that they are helping in some small way."

Her: "They help in a BIG way. They are my daily affirmation and motivation. I read and re-read them everyday."

That kind of blew me away and made me feel very good about my contribution. Still, I've found that she's on my mind constantly, and as a result this trip has been less joyful than previous ones.

Her prognosis is very good, and she lucked into one of the best oncologists in the city. I also hooked her up with my naturopath / acupuncturist - he's doing wonders with her mental outlook.

While I am very much looking forward to my couple of days on Oahu (and at the Kahala Resort!) I am also looking forward to getting home to provide more direct support.

I hope you have a good trip to Japan and I will see you the next time I'm in town.

2/17/12 - Insanely Proud Of You

I've tried to find the words to describe how proud I am of you for getting to the halfway point. For once, the nouns and verbs are not falling into the right places.

I cannot possibly tell you how much admiration I have for you - you've borne so much that I cannot imagine. But you are still standing. You're still here. Herman is a husk of his former self, and you are killing him every day. You have not backed down an inch, no matter how you've felt. You are winning.

The awfulness of my music collection is well known. Even then, every so often even a blind squirrel finds a nut.

On the other hand, I've listened to and watched this more times than I can count over the years. It is an amazing piece of music and message - I have no idea why more people don't know about it.

Watch it, sing it, live it.

"I've lived to see the sun break through the storm. I'm so glad to be standing here today."

I love you and believe in you. You're going to see the sun break through the storm.

http://www.youtube.com/watch?v=o6yD_LM2ch0&feature=youtube_gdata_player

(If the link doesn't work, Google "Joe Cocker I'm so glad to be standing here today" (without the quotes) and pick the top result.)

PS - Besides, the other option was Bon Jovi's "Living on a prayer" for the lyric "Oh...we're halfway there". Trust me - this one is way better.

2/18/12 - Here's To The Killers of Herman:

Here's to the killers of Herman, The doctors. The friends. The family. And most importantly Carla - the One True Big C.

The ones who conspire to commit murder on a malevolent 15 centimeter centipede.

They ignore the rules, they cheat, they bring him pain. They comfort, they inspire, they irradiate, and they have one focus - killing him.

Herman can groan and whine as he is dying, about the unfairness of being ganged up on.

About the only thing Herman can't do is ignore them. Because they're everywhere. They're the ones that bring the food to sustain the Big C. They're the ones that deliver the poison he's bathing in, or the inspiration that makes her stronger.

And while Herman may see them as murderers, as trained killers, we see genius.

Because Carla is stronger than she ever knew. Herman messed with the wrong hardass, and he is going down.

I love and believe in you. Believe in yourself. You're doing this, and you're winning. Use this weekend to restore your strength, to get ready to finish him. I'm so incredibly proud of you and cannot wait to see you on Monday.

2/19/12 - Adding Another Support Pillar

Well, I have returned, and I'm so very happy to be back in Seattle, for lots of reasons, but chief among them is that another pillar gets added to your support team in more than the passive way that I've participated in the past 3 weeks.

3 weeks. Hard to believe that you're halfway done. I really can't imagine how difficult it has been for you, but you've gotten the job done so far, just as I knew you were capable of doing.

Hearing that you were up and around today made me feel so good for you. You've earned the right to have good days, even as Herman's days get progressively worse. 15 cm of malevolence simply cannot stand up to the things that you've put him through.

I am so excited to be able to see you tomorrow and take you to visit with The Naturopath. As many times as I have seen him, I think of the appointments less as treatment and more as visits. And I'm excited to finally talk to you in person, to tell you how much I admire your spirit and your strength and your resolve.

Herman has none of those things. He doesn't have Stu and your sister and your friends and your med team and The Naturopath and myself, plus everyone else on the peripheries of things. He will collapse because he has none of those things. You will prevail because you have all of those things, plus you have you and everything you are, which is all you really need. Your will is Unbreakable. You are Unbreakable.

We all love and believe in you, and as usual, you've exceeded everyone's expectations.

I'll see you around 3 on Monday.

2/20/12 - Mirth

OK, I've never had a good poker face, and not being able to see you in person for the last several weeks allowed my imagination to run wild. I've been operating mainly on faith for this time.

My faith has been rewarded.

You look great, as your sister assured me that you would, but the thing that convinced me that you're winning is not the look in your eyes after you came out of the appointment with The Naturopath

It was the look before.

I'm not sure how to describe what I saw. Resolve and Strength come to mind, but there was more than those facile adjectives. It took me a while to pin it down, but I think I finally figured out what it is. Mirth.

You've always had a playful nature - I was worried that this experience had taken it out of you. If anything, I saw it burning even more brightly.

Call it what you will, but your Carla-ness is shining through. Whatever it is in your basic essence that makes you you, it has finally bubbled to the surface (or perhaps some layers have been peeled away). In another context, I would say that you're glowing.

I've never been more convinced that you are going to win this in a big way - not just surviving, but thriving. I've been writing on faith for the past 3 weeks, and now I've seen that I placed my faith in the right place.

Nobody comes into your house and pushes you around, according to the movie Rudy.

Keep pushing. Keep turning the corner. Keep rolling Herman back. Enjoy the small miracles that you've seen since you were diagnosed. Use the life force that you've tapped into.

Enjoy every minute where there are no cramps, because Herman is still under constant assault.

I love you and I'm thrilled to see that my continued Belief in you has been rewarded.

2/21/12 - No Compromises

Herman got more than he bargained for when he decided to take up residence in your nether regions. From Goodfellas:

Now the guy's got Carla as a partner. Any problems, he goes to Carla. Trouble with the bill? He can go to Carla. Trouble with the cops, deliveries, Tommy, he can call Carla. But now the guy's gotta come up with Carla's money every week, no matter what. Business bad? Fuck you, pay me. Oh, you had a fire? Fuck you, pay me. Place got hit by lightning, huh? Fuck you, pay me.

(later)

And then finally, when you can't borrow another buck from the bank, you bust the joint out. You light a match.

Herman wrote a check that as it turns out he can't pay for. He messed with the wrong person. Oh? Bathing in poison? Fuck you, pay me. Oh? Being burned by radiation? Fuck you. Pay me.

He can't come up with the money. Light a match.

Herman is a Dead Tumor Walking.

Early on in WWII, the Allies adopted a policy: nothing less than unconditional surrender from Germany, Italy, and Japan. Unconditional surrender is a tall order.

This was adopted primarily as a reaction to the problems that arose after World War One, and the Allies stuck to it.

No fucking compromises. Do not yield, and accept nothing less than unconditional surrender. When he is down, keep kicking him. You have Herman on the run.

I'm insanely happy to hear today's results. In retrospect, it seems silly for me to have worried about how you would look when I saw you. Your eyes gave it away immediately - you're the same Carla I've always known. In a strange way, you're a better Carla than I have known in a very long time.

At the same time, this is not your chance to rest on your laurels. Punish Herman. Harry him. Nip at his heels.

Keep up the skeer. Even when it doesn't matter any more.

You can do this. You've already done it. They can't scare you any more. They've tried, but they cannot possibly get to you.

Time to go on the offensive, courtesy of The Matrix.

Tank: So what do you need? Besides a miracle.

Neo: Guns. Lots of guns.

Trinity: Neo... nobody has ever done this before.

Neo: That's why it's going to work.

Lots of people have done this before, and you have access to lots of metaphorical guns.

Faced with an implacable foe? Fuck you. Pay me.

Be Unbreakable. Be Invincible. Destroy Herman.

2/22/12 - The Refrigerator

Everyone in America has their refrigerator moment - the time when they were 6 or 7 years old and came home from Kindergarten, usually with one or two teeth missing, bearing whatever horrifically bad art they had created.

They presented their treasure to their parent(s), these godlike creatures who knew how to cook things and were the source of everything.

The godlike creatures would smile at crayon drawings that were completely indecipherable, and then they would find room on the refrigerator for their newest creations.

If their experience was anything like mine, they would be filled with pride - "I did that", they would think.

Years later, I've seen enough of human behavior to say definitively that we all still seek the refrigerator moment. The moment where your effort and ingenuity is posted for the world to see. You and I often joke about the fact that most of life after high school is a replay of high school, and there is some truth to that.

But what we are really looking for as adults is a repeat of the refrigerator moment.

I have been insanely lucky in my life - I left a company that told me that selling metals on the Internet would never work. I went out and made it work. They realized their error and bought us. That was my refrigerator moment. I DID THIS!

This is a refrigerator moment for you. I remember the look on your face and in your eyes when you said "this will be the hardest thing I've ever done."

There was a level of resignation in that statement. But you've done it. You've lived to see the sun break through the clouds. This is a refrigerator moment. Even though you still have time left doing it, you can legitimately say:

I DID THIS.

Nobody can ever take this away from you. Here's the best part - after you've done this, there is nothing you can't do. You've discovered an inner toughness that you had only hinted at in the past.

Enjoy your refrigerator moment. You've earned it. And then start planning for the life you live after that. You have greatness in you. Let it flow out of you.

I love you and support you.

2/23/12 - Go That Way

Got a little too drunk tonight, so I don't have any awesome quotes. All I can tell you is that you've done more than anyone could have expected you to do.

It was gratifying to see the look in your eyes a couple of days ago, and to hear your voice through the door of The Naturopath's office. Unlike the spoon, you have not bent. You are carving your own path.

This is what people like you do. I've tried to measure myself against people like you, and I invariably come up wanting.

This will come to an end, and soon Herman will be a distant memory, vanquished if by nothing else than the force of your will. The whole world is open to you, because you have no fear.

Take the next step into a wider world. Only you can define what that step is. Go out there and take it.

I love you and support you.

2/24/12 (Part I) - Good Morning!

Wow. Went a little bit over the edge last night. Did not expect that.

I know that this is out of the normal order, but I've been thinking a lot lately about how difficult this must be for you and I want you to know just how much admiration that I have for what you're doing, and for the fact that what I saw on Monday - the look in your eyes - the sparkle that I've always known, is still there.

I can't possibly imagine how you must feel right now, but I hope that you can take some solace in the fact that everyone around you is thinking about you and hoping and praying for you, even people that you've never met, like my Uncle Chuck and Aunt Kazuko. You are getting better, even though it may not feel like it from moment to moment. Please try to remember that.

We all love and support you.

2/24/12 (Part II) - Not Sure About A Subject

I really hope that this note finds you well. For once, it will be brief.

You're the best thing that has ever happened to me.

If I could figure out a way to take this away from you, I would. I can only offer the fact that I and a large number of people love you and believe in you.

If there is anything that you need, please ask. No matter how small or large, we are here to help you.

2/24/12 (Part III) -

My heart goes out to you. You're in my thoughts all the time - I'm just happy that I'm able to help in some way.

If you need anything at all, just let me know. I'm a terrible cook, but I probably couldn't screw up soup too badly, and I am very good with scrambled eggs. I'm also available for runs to Jack In The Box for chicken sandwiches.

Everything that I've read keeps coming back to one thing - while this is hard on you, it is way harder on Herman, and the docs aren't doing anything that will permanently hurt you. This is temporary and transitory and it will end soon. You are getting better.

You've shown an awful lot of grit and I am immensely proud of you. Keep breathing and don't be afraid to ask the universe for a little help. I love you and support you.

Text Messages: 2/25/12 9:53 AM

Me: Feeling better today?

Carla: No the final stretch has unique challenges. Been having bad dizzy spells and almost passing out. Something new to deal with. Fun times.

Me: Be well, Carla. You're almost through. Herman's going down. Can I get you anything?

Carla: Thanks for the offer but all I can do is stay in bed and try to build my strength. Broing but I need a lot of rest this weekend. The next two weeks will be the hardest yet, so here we go!!

2/25/12 - Time Flies

I was thinking about something I heard a long time ago about how time seems to accelerate as we age. A year suddenly doesn't seem as long as it used to.

When we were kids, the 2 weeks before Christmas might as well have been 5 years - they stretched out so far in front of us and it never seemed like it would get here. Of course, we were also being bored to death in school, so there is that factor to consider.

Most Decembers now fly by. OLM is two quarters into our fiscal year, and it feels like the last one just ended.

The phenomenon is based on the simple fact that when we were 10, a year was 10% of our total life experience - all the things that took place in a year then filled a huge portion of our experience bank.

At this point in our lives, a year represents a little more than 2% of the time since we were born, and with each passing day, any individual day represents a smaller percentage of your life.

There are 12 days left before your Christmas and New Year's Day and other major/minor holidays, when they take out the chemo pack and take X-rays to show you what you've managed to do to Herman.

This represents 0.06% of your life experience.

These 12 days will be some of the more difficult ones that you've had. But they represent a smaller and smaller number of days that you'll have to do this. And you've proven your toughness, that you can do this, with everything that has been thrown at you.

When it becomes difficult, think of Louie from Unbroken and his time in the raft. He had no idea when or even if it would ever end. You have a date that you can look forward to, when you know this will be over. This will end.

Remember what The Naturopath said as you were telling him the story of your diagnosis - "And they were as surprised as you were." You are fundamentally healthy and your body can handle this.

You are far tougher than you can ever imagine, as long as you Believe. Believe that you can get through it, and you will.

You can do this, Carla. I love you deeply and support you.

2/26/12 - The Watershed Line

You're going to read Cryptonomicon by Neal Stephenson if I have to email it to you 3 paragraphs at a time. Kidding. Ok, not really.

There's one section that seems really appropriate to where you are right now. Bear with me:

"Imagine this, Waterhouse. The emperor is meeting with his general staff. All of the top generals and admirals in Nippon parade into the room in full dress uniforms and bow down solemnly before the emperor. They have come to report on the progress of the war. Each of these generals and admirals is wearing a brand-new hachimaki around his forehead. These hachimakis are printed with phrases saying things like 'through my personal incompetence I killed two hundred thousand of our own men' and 'I handed our Midway plans over to Nimitz on a silver platter.'

"See, we've gone over the watershed line in this war. We won Midway. We won North Africa. We won Stalingrad. The Battle of the Atlantic. Everything changes when you go over the watershed line. The rivers all flow a different direction. It's as if the force of gravity itself has changed and is now working in our favor."

The point here is that you have passed the watershed line. All of the rivers are flowing downhill. The force of gravity has changed in your favor.

The metaphor even extends fairly well when you consider where it happens in the novel - the war was effectively over, but the campaigns for the Philippines, Iwo Jima, and Okinawa were still to come. Japan was defeated - they just didn't know it yet.

Your war is all but over - there are several hard battles to fight, but the outcome is not in doubt any more. You will emerge from this the victor. Herman is done. His time is through. And it is all because of the strength and toughness that is innate to who you are. That has never changed, and it has never been in doubt.

Rely on it. It is your gift, it is your talent. It will see you through.

I love you unconditionally and support you, no matter what you need. Keep getting better.

2/27/12 - It Has Been In You Along

I don't even know where to start after our call - we covered a lot of ground.

Ok, let's start with this - your faith and belief is being rewarded. The fact that you can eat (and pass) a lot of different foods is evidence of your increasing dominance over Herman. Fuck the marker numbers. He's shrinking. Digestion is proof of your dominance.

It isn't over, of course, but you're over the watershed line. The rivers have changed course. It will get easier. It will get better. The pain will end.

You have been proven to be far tougher than you ever imagined. Rely on that. You will still have your fuck fuck fuck moments, but you've proven that you're bigger than that. You've done this, and you can do it again.

In Drago-speak: you are a piece of iron.

I wanted to comment on something you said tonight, but I was still short of material and so I held back. You were talking about how your relationship with your sister has become so much deeper via this trip through hell.

My thought was this - it is a shame that this experience is what it takes to discover these feelings. You talked about the joyful moments. I love the fact that you see the positive arising from what you've gone through.

Lest we end on a down note - the ability to do this has been within you all along. Cancer has not discovered something new. Rely upon your basic nature, upon who you were before being diagnosed.

It has been in you all along.

Text Messages: 2/28/12 4:20 PM

Me: Really happy to hear that the days have gotten a little easier to make it through. You've earned it.

Carla: That's not what I'm saying at all. They are hard, fucking hard. Right now I can't move because of the pain. Oh no not easier, I am just getting thru it!

Me: You're the toughest person I know. Not much time left. This will end. Not soon enough, but it will end.

Me: I'm proud of you, but more importantly you should be proud of yourself. You're doing this!

Carla: I'm in too much pain to feel much of anything. Sorry to be so blunt I'm just feeling pretty bad right now. Wish I could be more positive at this moment. Just can't do it. Sorry.

Me: I know. I'm wishing you nothing but the best.

Carla: Thanks. If you could wish death to Herman that would be helpful too.

Me: Been doing that the entire time. Looking into voodoo to polish him off.

2/28/12 (Part I) - Time Has Little To Do With Infinity And Jelly Doughnuts

I'm a little early with tomorrow's email, but I am not above cheating when necessary. The ends justify the means.

Ok, we've got two options here. Never thought that my life-long obsession with Magnum would come in this handy.

Herman is Magnum-based, so he is susceptible to two episodes - Home From The Sea (Season 4) and Limbo (the last episode of Season 7). The title of this email actually derives from the first episode of Season 8.

Let's go with the more straightforward version first. Magnum finds himself knocked off of his surfski and drifting in the ocean. He is bumped by a shark, and remembers when he was a kid and scared of monsters. His dad tells him to name the monster, and Herman was born.

In this episode, Magnum tells Herman that he wants to play hide-and-go seek, and Herman gets to hide first. He closes his eyes, counts to ten, and when he opens his eyes, Herman is gone. Closing our eyes and counting to ten is not really that effective of a chant, so we'll set that aside for a moment.

In Limbo, Magnum is shot and lies in a coma for most of the episode. Except for the gunshot wound, he is, like you, fundamentally healthy, but he is slipping away.

Rick: "We've tried everything."

Higgins: "Unless...we've overlooked the obvious."

Higgins marches into Magnum's room, comes to attention, and in his best Sergeant-Major's voice, says: "Magnum, I demand you come back here immediately."

Magnum flatlines soon thereafter in order to create a cliffhanger for the 8th season.

In the 8th season premiere, Magnum has to make a choice, and he comes back due to some unfinished business. He's pronounced dead, and 15 seconds thereafter sits up, looks around, and says "A pint of stout. I'd like a pint of stout."

This ties back into something from the previous episode - Higgins told a story about a miraculous recovery he had witnessed where one of his fellow soldiers had been pronounced dead, and then sat up, looked around, and asked for a pint of stout.

Ok, so lots of geeky Magnum worship here. Of all the things you know about me, I think that this is the most embarrassing. And that is a pretty high bar.

Anyway, we have the basis for a chant. The first part must be delivered with an English accent. When you're doing it, say it like it is written. When other people are doing it, substitute the word "her" for "here".

Again, best British Sergeant-Major voice:

"Herman! I demand you leave here immediately!"

Accent not required for the second part:

"...the bar is closed and we're out of stout. You don't have to go home but you can't stay here."

Be well, Carla. I love you and support you.

2/28/12 (Part II) - YAYG

Consider this the bonus round. I'm really not in control of my muse - it happens when it happens, and I've learned to pay attention when an idea pops into my head.

One of the Fox's favorite abbreviations was YAYG. You Ask, You Get. For the neanderthals in the steel industry that he was selling to, it meant that the piece of paper in their inbox would seamlessly move to their outbox, and that no problems would occur with their shipments that would inconvenience them.

There is a larger lesson here - call it God, or the Universe, at work. I'm not smart enough to distinguish between the two, or the One, depending upon your point of view.

YAYG does not work if you're wishing for a billion dollars. If you're asking for the toughness to get through a difficult afternoon, it has a better than average chance of working.

The Naturopath and I were talking about Steve Jobs' last words, which were reported as "oh wow, wow, wow." I interpreted that as his last message - there is something beyond us.

The Naturopath the scientist actually disappointed me by telling me that at the moment of passing, the body dumps a whole lot of awesome chemicals into the bloodstream - Jobs' experience was not unique.

But then I started thinking about it - there is exactly zero reason, from a biological/genetic selection perspective, for the release of all the good-feeling chemicals. This basic set of facts has made me crazy for a week or so.

As Benjamin Franklin said, "beer is proof that God loves us and wants us to be happy."

There is something else out there. I don't know what to call it, but I suspect that every so often it will provide a tail wind for those that have earned it.

You've earned it.

So ask for some relief. Ask that Herman has been vanquished. Ask that the bar is closed, and they're out of stout.

I don't know the combination, and have only had fleeting glimpses of something larger than what we see, but I have become more and more convinced that it is there. The worst case when you ask for help is that none comes, and you're no worse off.

The bar is closed, Herman. You don't have to go home, but you can't stay here.

Keep the faith, Carla. You can do this. Ask for a tailwind whenever you need it, but recognize how tough you are. Be Unbreakable.

I love you and support you.

Text Messages: 2/29/12 3:01 PM

Me: Herman's leaving. Immediately. Hope you're doing ok today.

Carla: Keep that thought going. I know I do! Thanks for the awesome emails. Loved them both.

Me: You're doing awesome, Carla. He doesn't stand a chance.

2/29/12 - Renewable Resources

As you enter the final week of round one, I went back into the archives to see if there was anything I had missed, or anything I should have emphasized more.

One of the things that I talked about was tapping in to your reserves (this is different from tapping into something larger, which I've beaten like a dead horse.)

Do you remember the story about asking Fox for a tailwind? The coda to that story is that once I got to within about 2 miles of the end, I made the decision to not leave anything on the trail. After 24 miles, I sprinted the last 10% of the course, and I still had more left in my tank when my magnificent calves finished the trip.

It took me a while to figure out the message of Unbroken, once I got past my desire to smack every Japanese person within a 500-foot radius silly on general principles. It didn't help that there were like 7 Japanese tour groups within smacking distance for the entire trip.

What ties these two paragraphs together? Renewable resources.

We hear a lot about wind and solar as the ultimate renewable resources. You know different - you've tapped in to something personal that has sustained you throughout this ordeal. It isn't quantifiable. But it is there, and it exists within you. It will remain with you once you're done.

But here is the best part - not only are your own reserves nearly inexhaustible, they renew themselves on a regular basis. You couldn't have gotten this far if they didn't. They are recharging right now, even as they give you strength.

Rely on your reserves. That's what they are there for. Evolution has spent millions of years refining them. Don't worry about using them up - they will regenerate.

I love you and I support you - you can do this. You've already proven it. Breathe deeply - inhale bliss and exhale Herman.

March

(During a visit to the Naturopath, he was able to see the cramping for himself and immediately hooked her up to an IV. To this day, we still don't know what was in it. We just started calling it the Magic IV).

Text Messages: 3/1/12 8:56 PM

Carla: I will. So far starting to feel a bit better and no cramps. We will see how it works.

Me: Great news on no cramping.

Carla: Still cramp free so we may have found a winner. Fingers crossed.

Me: FUCK YEAH!

Carla: Still no cramps. This could be a fucking miracle.

3/1/12 - Random Thoughts

Let's call this a smorgasbord - no really central organizing theme, just a bunch of random thoughts.

- Re the marker going from 9 to 11 - how the fuck did we miss this part - "It goes to 11." No. It STOPS at 11.

- Switching to a second classic comedy movie - imagine Herman as the Black Knight in Holy Grail. Legless, armless, reduced to trying to bite the ankles of Sir Arthur.

And failing miserably. Herman has been neutered.

- Thrilled to hear that you experienced a relief from the cramping tonight. FUCK YEAH was as pure of a response as I could provide. Presuming that The Naturopath's Magic IV was the proximate cause of your relief, do not hesitate to call on The Naturopath, even when you don't have an appointment. What else is he doing - rearranging his furniture?

As I said a couple of days ago, I am not above cheating, and you know how I feel about cheating. If you need a resource, reach out to it. As Fox used to say - "What is your worst-case scenario?" In this instance, the worst case is that the resource is unavailable or says no.

That isn't going to happen - I'm better at reading people than most give me credit for - every single person I know who is involved with supporting you will do whatever it takes, and whatever you need, and I am pretty sure that includes The Naturopath. If you need it, find out.

- I'm glad I finally got to meet you at Group Health. Your comments about the tunnel, and the different feelings you get depending upon the direction that you're traveling, gave a lot of texture to the conversations we've had.

104

There is obviously a metaphor there; as it is, I'm just happy to have experienced it at least once.

- I'm equally grateful for the time we spent mocking the organic coffee shop people. More than anything, it told me that while you've been scarred by this, and your life has been irrevocably changed, your capacity for seeing stupidity, and your disdain for it, hasn't changed. We need more people like you in the world. For right now, it seems like we will have to be happy and treasure the ones that we have. You are treasured.

- I recall two quotes, from widely divergent sources, and I hope that you can meditate on them, because I think that they apply to the life you learn with and the life you live with after that.

First - the coach of the Steelers in the 1970's, Chuck Noll, was known for bringing players he was about to cut into his office and asking "what is your life's work?" The implication was that there is a whole world out there beyond football to conquer.

Second - even though it ended badly for both parties, the best recruiting line of all time belongs to Steve Jobs, when he was trying to lure a Pepsi executive to work at Apple - "Do you want to sell sugar water for the rest of your life, or do you want to come with me and change the world?"

I know that right now killing Herman is your only focus. Maybe you want to go back to the comfortable womb of your job at Garvey, and there isn't anything wrong with that, especially after what you've endured.

Still, stepping on to the high wire is what people like you and I are built for.

You've earned the right to not step on the wire again, but we both know that it isn't in our nature. You're not going to jump out of a plane physically, but I can't see you selling sugar water for the rest of your life either.

The whole world is open to you. You cannot be scared of anything any more. You've faced it. You've had more 3 am moments than I care to think about. There is power and magic and genius in your story.

- Finally, the relief from cramping tonight inspires me to commit plagiarism from The Princess Bride:

Inigo Montoya: You are wonderful.

Man in Black: Thank you; I've worked hard to become so.

Inigo Montoya: I admit it, you are better than I am.

Man in Black: Then why are you smiling?

Inigo Montoya: Because I know something you don't know.

Man in Black: And what is that?

Inigo Montoya: I... am not left-handed.

[Moves his sword to his right hand and gains an advantage]

Man in Black: You are amazing.

Inigo Montoya: I ought to be, after 20 years.

Man in Black: Oh, there's something I ought to tell you.

Inigo Montoya: Tell me.

Man in Black: I'm not left-handed either.

And now you're not left-handed either. DEATH TO HERMAN!

Text Messages: 3/2/12 2:17 AM

Carla: This is a miracle. I have other issues but the soul crushing pain is gone for tonight.

Me: So happy to wake up to this message. Don't be afraid to cheat and reach out for more as you close out phase one.

Carla: I had a decent night sleep and again no huge cramps. I did w not wake up except for small issues. I will see about getting another one next week I am so happy this morning.

(During the final week or so of her initial treatment, Carla was approached by one of the docs and told that Herman was definitely shrinking. This was huge news for all involved and gave her hope that perhaps the surgery would not be as extensive as she feared - there was a real chance that due to the size and the placement of Herman, she would be looking at a permanent, rather than temporary, colostomy.)

Text Messages: 3/2/12 3:26 PM

Carla: Only have a second. Tumor is definitely shrinking. Will update you latere.

Me: Awesome fucking news.

Carla: Call me when u can talk.

Carla: You're such a liar. You would be worried about me if I had split ends! I don't have split ends though. I have great hair!

Me: Ok. Now I'm no more worried than usual.

Carla: That's more like it!

3/2/12 - It Turns Out The Spoon Actually Does Bend

Ray Kinsella: What are you grinning at, you ghost?

Shoeless Joe Jackson: If you build it...

[nods toward John Kinsella]

Shoeless Joe Jackson: ... HE will come.

Ray Kinsella: Ease his pain...Go the distance...It was you...

Shoeless Joe Jackson: No, Ray. It was YOU.

I should probably leave it at that conversation from Field of Dreams, and let you connect the dots, but I can't. After all you've been through, I want to celebrate the one thing that got you to this point, the one thing that made it possible.

Today's jaw-dropping conversation with your doc has at its heart the fact that you were able to see it through - that you were able to tap into reserves that you didn't know existed - that you alone endured the 3 am moments for the past (I checked) 51 days. Jesus. That's a long fucking time.

In your private moments, the kind of moments that you don't talk about at parties, know that as much as there were lots of people helping, or trying to help, or getting in the way, this really came down to who you are. You haven't really changed that much from the person I've known all of these years, and that has made all of the difference. All of the support in the world wouldn't have meant jackshit if you weren't who you are.

That part was never really in doubt.

You were needed on that wall.

Take quiet pride in this moment. Close your eyes and remember the feeling. While the fight is not over, this was where, finally, the rivers started officially running in a different direction. Or at least where your docs let you have a peek at what your efforts have wrought and proved what we've known all along.

Today was your Neo moment, when he finally saw the Matrix in code - the world warped around him, and rather than him bending, the spoon gave way.

There is much left to do, and you will need to do it with as much intensity as you've prosecuted the war on Herman thus far. The difference now is that before you believed, and now you know.

Victory, it is said, has a thousand fathers. Lots of people helped you along the way. In the end, though...

No, Carla, it was YOU.

Oh, almost forgot - DEATH TO HERMAN!

3/3/12 - A Leap From The Lion's Head

Spent the afternoon watching Indiana Jones III - what a perfect movie.

"Only by a leap from the lion's head will the knight prove his worth."

You've made that leap, again and again and again. You've proven that you are worthy. Rest and store your energy. Herman isn't going out without a fight, however brief.

But he is going to lose. Instead of believing it, you know it. Keep up the skeer - punish him, harry him, nip at his heels. Force him into mistakes. Even when it doesn't matter any more.

No surrender. No mercy. You are a piece of iron.

Text Messages: 3/4/12 9:03 AM

Me: Hope last night went better for you. Would you be up for a visit later?

Carla: Chris. Honestly the pain is tremendous. Every night is harder than the last. I am sitting in the dark right now barley able to type this but at least it takes my mind off the pain and burning for a few minutes. I know and am so happy the say things are working but I can't feel it right now. I just keep holding out for this week.

Carla: This is so awful with only minutes of relief. Stu wanted me to go to the ER but I remind him everyday this is suppose to be normal. Norma!!

Carla: Just having a hard time believing today, ya know.

Carla: The pain is normal. They tell me that every week. The can only help me to manage it through the meds. The ER can't do anything. Trust me I got this down to an art. I'm just so very tired. Trying to handle the pain and kill a tumor takes all my energy.

Me: I'm starting to understand better. You're the gutsiest person I know, and you have all my love and support.

Carla: Thank you but trust me I don't think I'm gutsy at all. Most of the time I feel like a huge wimp.

Me: Don't sell yourself short. What you're doing is the definition of gutsy.

Carla: Thanks.

Me: You're welcome. Keep kicking his ass!

3/4/12 - This Week Is Your Week

I've spent a lot of time thinking about your last week of treatment, and all the soaring language I would use to inspire you.

Let's be honest, though. All that soaring language sounds like bullshit when you're fighting cramps and burns that seem like they will never end. Concepts are not operable at this level. Right now, it is nothing less than pure resolve that gets you through.

This will end, and I quote myself in saying that it will end sooner than you expect it to. You will have a long life, free of this scourge. You are killing Herman. You will emerge the victor.

I wanted to address something you said today, that you felt like a wimp. Nothing could be further from the truth. You've taken this head-on, and borne the burden. You are the epitome of guts, and nobody can ever say otherwise. You are a piece of iron.

I know I have a Galahad complex - you identified it in me years ago. I want to preserve and protect those who are close to me. It has been especially active lately for obvious reasons.

Our conversations today via text reminded me of that, but it also gave me an insight that I want you to consider.

This week is Carla Time. This week is the time that all of your essence is focused on killing Herman, or dealing with the ramifications of killing Herman.

You and I are so similar it is scary - if I were dealing with anything close to this, I would be worrying that I wasn't at

113

work and contributing. I get that on a deeper level than you might imagine.

But this time is for you. This time is to let your body do what it is capable of to send Herman home in a body bag. I understand that you're frustrated by not being able to do the things you used to be able to do. Trust me, I get it. It is ok to focus in on just this. It is ok to let go.

Work will be there when you're done with this. Right now, take care of yourself - give yourself permission to be as selfish as an 8 year old with a cold.

The stakes are higher, but the basic principle is the same. Your team will take care of you. (There is, of course, a remote chance that we will mock you later. We are not saints. Forgive us). I really hope you know I'm kidding about this part. Seriously - totally kidding!!!

If you need something, say it. Don't ask, don't demand. It will be provided. This is what we are here for - unconditionally. Let us take care of you.

This is Carla Week. You have our unconditional love and support and permission to be as selfish as you need to be.

Basically, this is the best birthday week ever. You ask, you get. This is your time. Herman's time is through.

You're the toughest person I know. You have proven that you are not a wimp.

A long time ago, when I was first learning to play golf, I did something that a lot of people who are new to the game do - I kept trying to help the ball into the air. The result was that I kept hitting the top of the ball and doing the exact opposite of what I was trying to do - the ball would skitter down the fairway and end up 50 yards away, rather than 150 yards.

Finally, Fox pulled me aside and explained how the shape of the clubs had been designed by people with very large brains who were paid to do nothing else other than to build clubs that would get the ball into the air.

They had taken the work out of it. All you had to do was to rely on the fact that the designers knew what they were doing.

Whether you choose to believe in God or not, there is no denying (unless you are a whacko Evangelical Christian and have hidden that fact from me for over a decade) that the process of evolution over a million or so years has provided our bodies with remarkable tools.

One of those tools that we've provided ourselves is the capacity to heal. It is in us. Every single one of us. It is in you. Let your body do the work. It is your ally.

In yet another attempt to get you to read Cryptonomicon 3 paragraphs at a time:

"Let's set the existence-of-God issue aside for a later volume, and just stipulate that in some way, self-replicating organisms came into existence on this planet and immediately began trying to get rid of each other, either by spamming their environments with rough copies of themselves, or by more direct means which hardly need be belabored. Most of them failed, and their genetic legacy was erased from the universe forever, but a few found some way to propagate. After about three billion years...

"...Laurence Pritchard Waterhouse was born. Laurence was, by birthright, a stupendous badass, in that he could trace his ancestry back up a long line of slightly less highly evolved stupendous badasses to that first self-replicating gizmo - which, given the number and variety of its descendants, might justifiably be described as the most stupendous badass of all time.

Everyone and everything that wasn't a stupendous badass was dead."

You are a stupendous badass. This next week is your week. I love and support you in all that you do.

Be well, Carla. Be selfish, and feel zero guilt about it. This is your time. This week is your week.

Also - DEATH TO HERMAN!!!

Text Messages: 3/5/12 7:05 PM

Me: These next three will be love taps compared to what you have gutted your way through, and then it is done.

Me: Be selfish, rest, and let your body heal itself.

Carla: No I don't think so. Today was the worst day so far. I'm in unbelievable pain and taking all of the pills and pot I can stand.

Me: This will end. My heart goes out to you. It is almost over, and it will pass.

Me: You're strong enough to do this.

3/5/12 - Goethe

I was kind of drifting, looking for a theme or a hook for tonight's message. I even asked Fox for a tailwind.

Then it struck me - the Antarctic Explorer guy that you were so freaked out about introducing back in 1999. The beginning of Carla 2.0. The start of my personal path. The message I left, in binary code, when my first stint at Copper & Brass was at an end. Amazing how so many things can happen at the same time. There are precisely zero coincidences.

Do you remember how he opened up his presentation?

"If you can dream it or do it, begin now, for boldness has magic and power and genius in it."
- Goethe

This is the birth of Carla 3.0 - a more elegant weapon, for a less civilized age.

You're not quite there yet - you have some other things on your mental roster of things to do, like "STOPPING THIS PAIN IN MY GUT" and "STOPPING THIS HORRIFIC SUNBURN", and "ok, the cramping was interesting at the beginning and now I fit into a size 2, but FUCKING ENOUGH ALREADY."

This is the beginning of the end. You've done everything right. Just as importantly, you've done it well.

Tiny steps for the next couple of days. Be selfish - we are all here to take care of you. Absolutely unconditional. You say, you get.

But Carla 3.0 is waiting to be born. I know you - in many ways I am you. You have a higher purpose. You have some time to decide what it is.

Best recruiting line of all time - "do you want to sell sugar water for the rest of your life, or do you want to come with me and change the world?"

You can keep selling sugar water, and enjoy a fine existence. But that isn't in your nature. Your future is not fixed.

Time has little to do with infinity and jelly donuts.

Trust me on the last part.

In the meantime, begin now.

(I don't remember the guy's name, but Carla's firm brought in an Antarctic explorer who started off his speech with the Goethe quote. I was so impressed that when I left my old job before I joined OnlineMetals I sent an all-company email with the quote translated into binary. So, so geeky. It also led to a wholesale review of who had access to all-company email addresses, which is always fun.)

Text Messages: 3/6/12 11:45 PM

Me: Hard to believe that this phase is almost over. Look at what a stupendous badass you've shown yourself to be.

Me: Sleep well, Carla. Sleep well.

Carla: Thank you and although I am up at this early hour I will be back to sleep soon. Had a good night last night.

3/6/12 - Wars End

From the criminally unappreciated HBO series The Wire:

Kima: You rogue motherfuckers kill me. Fighting the war on drugs, one brutality case at a time.

Carver: You can't call this shit a war.

Herc: Why not?

Carver: Wars end.

This would seem like an unlikely entry point for today's email - they're talking about a war without end, and phase one of your war is almost done. I can't help myself - I came across a site that had the 100 best quotes from The Wire, and that one really struck me.

Do not go Googling it - you haven't seen the entire series, so a lot of them will be out of context. In addition, I don't want you to spoil things if you ever decide to watch it all, WHICH YOU SHOULD, AND I MAY MAKE YOU. Finally, as a Wire snob, you haven't earned the right yet.

Yes, I am aware that I am telling my best friend, who spent the better part of the last two months in a battle with cancer, that she hasn't earned that right yet. That's how seriously I take this.

Ok, now that I am done being self-indulgent and depressing, which is the opposite of why I started writing to you, let's talk about something more germane:

Wars do end.

As I write this, you are 39 hours and 51 minutes away from completing phase one. There has been nothing about this that has been easy, but you have done it. The obvious thing is to say that, as Jimmy from A League of Their Own pointed out, "it is the hard that makes it great", but that is facile Hollywood bullshit.

It is the hard that makes it hard.

I can't imagine how difficult this has been, and even though it will begin to ebb soon, it was still insanely hard. It would be nice if there was a medal for ordinary people who have borne extraordinary burdens.

900+ hours of chemo and radiation, according to the app on my phone. Fuck. You are my newest hero.

But you are still standing (more or less), and Herman is all but dead. You have done this.

You've done everything that could reasonably be expected of you. You've gone beyond what could reasonably be expected of you. You have nothing left to prove.

This war will end. The reason that it will end? Because you are tougher than Herman. Because your sister is there to exhibit her mom-ness. Because you have friends who spend way too much of their lives figuring out soup recipes.

You have an army behind you. As I said on day one, you have to do this by yourself, but you don't have to do it alone.

I love and support you - take care of yourself, Carla.

3/7/12 - Welcome to Day 0

There is a zen koan (puzzle/riddle/meditation aid) that goes:

Imagine that a baby goose has been placed inside a large bottle - some time later, the goose has grown too large for the bottle. How do you get the goose out of the bottle without either breaking the bottle or killing the goose?

The answer is simple: "There. It's out!"

I've had a hard time with this one over the years. First, the premise never made sense. Who the hell puts a baby goose in a bottle? Second, the answer, which is designed to confuse the person meditating and open them up to different ways of thinking, makes no fucking sense whatsoever.

I only have come to realize lately that we are the goose in the bottle. Artificial restrictions, whether societal or familial or whatever, are all around us. When we were still young, we had a chance of escaping them easily.

But the thing is - they're artificial. They don't really exist. Hence the answer - once you stop acknowledging that the bottle exists, the goose is out and unharmed.

Welcome to day 0. You've done it. You've done what you described as the "hardest thing you'll ever do." It isn't over, of course - this is only the first phase. It is, arguably, the most important one - you've stopped Herman in his tracks. You've shrunken him. You've cut him. He's not a machine. He's mortal.

You've counted to 10 and told him to go away.

And more than that, you have proven to yourself just what you are capable of. If you are capable of enduring this, of bearing the unbearable, think about this - although it is expressed many ways (what goes up must come down, etc.) - there is an immutable physical law:

For every action there is an equal, and opposite reaction.

Protons and electrons - equal and opposite. The reasons that rockets work are directly tied to this law. I could go on for hours.

The point is that for all of the ugliness that you've had to deal with in this ordeal, as you've told me there have been moments of joy. There is an equal and opposite reaction - you've shown a tremendous capacity to deal with pain and fear. Today is the first day that you start to explore how much happiness and optimism you can experience.

Think about the depths that you've gone through - the 500 yards of shit-smelling foulness that I can't even imagine, or maybe I don't want to.

(Relax. I'm not talking about farting. I love farts. Fart is the second funniest word in the English language after "poop". True story – my ex-wife had me convinced for the first 18 months of our relationship that girls don't fart. I made her pay for that with a whole lot of Dutch Ovens. But that is for another day. I'm talking metaphorically here.)

There is an equal and opposite reaction - you can experience happiness and peace at a level commensurate with where you found yourself during the darkest days of agony and fear. It is out there.

Andy Dufresne in The Shawshank Redemption: Get busy living, or get busy dying.

This is day zero. Time to decide what you're going to get busy doing.

Choose wisely, and welcome to the first day of the rest of your life.

This last part doesn't work perfectly, but it is so good, and so appropriate that I didn't feel that changing the pronouns was a good idea. Imagine yourself addressing Herman. Obviously, you are Neo from The Matrix.

"I know you're out there. I can feel you now. I know that you're afraid... you're afraid of us.

"You're afraid of change. I don't know the future. I didn't come here to tell you how this is going to end. I came here to tell you how it's going to begin.

"I'm going to hang up this phone, and then I'm going to show these people what you don't want them to see. I'm going to show them a world without you.

"A world without rules and controls, without borders or boundaries. A world where anything is possible.

"Where we go from there is a choice I leave to you."

Congratulations on doing what had to be done. There was nothing about it that was easy, but you did it. You've earned this, and for the rest of your life you never have to prove anything to anyone, even though we both know that it is in your nature to keep proving yourself.

The hard may in fact make it great.

I love and support you in all that you do. Be well, Carla. Be well.

Text Messages: 3/8/12 8:30 AM

Carla: So happy today is here!!

Me: Can't stop looking at the countdown clock. So incredibly proud of you.

Carla: Thank you and thank you for everything. I'm so glad this day has finally come!!

3/8/12 - A New Hope

What do you say to your best friend, who has just endured the unendurable? Are words sufficient to capture just how proud/happy/relieved/thrilled that I am for you?

No, they are not.

You fucking faced Herman down in the middle of the street and outgunned, outthought, outfought and outlasted him. Words can't do justice to that. Words can't express 10 weeks of 3 am moments for you.

I salute you. You did it. You are an inspirational figure. As I said last night, all the Hollywood bullshit aside, sometime the hard does make it great. You've touched greatness. You've lived and breathed it.

On Day One, I told you something - that it was your last day of playing defense against Herman. That day was the day you went on the offensive. Slowly but surely, you have gained the upper hand.

There is a Pacific War analogue to that moment, but explaining all the stuff that led up to it would take more time than I have, and you would likely fall asleep halfway through. Suffice it to say, it was big and important. Think the explosion of the Death Star in Star Wars IV. The rivers started to run the other way.

Now the rivers are flowing at maximum strength, eating away at Herman. You are growing stronger every minute of every day.

I know that you want to get back to some semblance of an ordinary life, but I urge you to take the time to let your body heal. Do not succumb to pressure from work, or from any other quarter, to rush back in. There is nothing to be gained from going back in too soon.

Work will still be there when you get back.

The comparison isn't equal, by any means, but I could spend about a week listing the number of football players who ended their careers by attempting to play too quickly after suffering a Dreaded High Ankle Sprain.

That's an injury that everyone knows takes a minimum of 6 weeks to come back from, even though the ankle feels good after 4 weeks and they try to come back, only to re-injure that same ankle. Then they're not right until 12-14 weeks later. The number of fantasy football seasons that have been wasted by the high ankle sprain is insanely large.

Take this time for yourself. Be selfish. Do not rush back in because you think people expect you to. Because when you decide to flip the switch on Carla 3.0, I want you to be at your absolute peak.

Carla 2.0 was a trained killer. Carla 2.0 was Jason Bourne.

I'm microwaving popcorn, and looking forward to the unveiling of Carla 3.0 - but I'm happy to wait for that until you're really ready to go.

I love you, I am thrilled that you made it to this day, and I can't wait to see what is next for you.

Just make sure that you are healed before you go off storming the castle.

3/8/12 - Letter to Family / Friends

Today was a big day - the last day of chemo and radiation. The end to nearly 800 hours of ranging between drug-induced stupor and unparalleled agony.

The docs have told her that Herman is retreating, but they won't say by how much. For right now, this is enough. It has to be.

And now we wait - the treatment will continue to work for the next month or so - her next appointment for tests is in 4 weeks, when they will learn (and hopefully tell her) the results of all the cramping and burning and sleepless nights.

Her ability to tap into her reserves, reserves she never knew existed, has been both remarkable and life-affirming. I know that if I am ever facing something like this, I will draw on my experience of watching her quiet strength and toughness.

Thanks for your support, whether overt or not, during this. It has been noticed and felt.

3/9/12 - Day 2 of Freedom

I don't have a whole lot of new stuff for you tonight, other than to emphasize that you are winning. Nobody expected this to be easy, and it has lived up to that part of the marketing brochure.

But you've done it. You've taken the worst that Herman can do. He's an evil little fucker, but he is dying, and you are the cause. You stood up to him. You have done this.

Let the medicine and your will do the rest.

I love you and I support you - you're going to do this!

Text Messages: 3/10/12 8:35 AM

Me: The healing is going on all the time. You body is repairing itself.

Carla: I'm such a friggin mess

Me: You're a wonderful, beautiful, stupendous badass who is killing Herman with each breath.

Carla: Thank you. He is puttng up a fight. Especially today.

Carla: Thanks so much for the awesome sweatpants. What did you do, buy out the store? Oh ya I think you did. I love them and so need them, especially for the next couple of weeks. Thank you again. Glad you could come and visit for a few. Maybe now you can understand how hard it is for me to have company. Anyway so glad to see you! And thanks for making everything with the juice company right!! I love you.

Me: I love you too. Happy to help in any way.

3/10/12 - Thank You

I'll keep this short - I know that you're tired, and that concentrating on a 4,000 word email is a little bit much right now.

First, thank you so much for letting me come in today, not once, but twice. It means a lot to me on more levels than you will ever likely know.

Second, and way more important to you - I can see and feel that you are winning. How? I can't put a finger on it - I just know it, in the same very deep way that I knew OnlineMetals would work out.

Your inner spark has not been diminished - whatever makes Carla Carla is still there. You're tired and sore, but look at where you were a week ago - tired and hurting and sore and burning.

You're making progress every single day, and that progress is accelerating. Right now it is baby steps, like being able to sleep through the night.

But those steps will accumulate - soon there will be an avalanche of good stuff that makes the last 2 months worthwhile. Or at least makes up for them.

Ok, I went way longer than I wanted to - sleep well, wake up well, be well. You have my unconditional love and support.

3/11/12 - First Steps

I'm going to keep these short until you tell me to crank things up again, and also because with the toughest part behind you, there isn't a need for the high-intensity coaching/inspiring stuff that I have been sending.

Here's what I'm seeing - you may not see the changes because they're happening gradually to you, but with more time between visits, the changes are more obvious.

Yesterday you could barely stand. Today you were walking around. Slowly, but you were still walking around.

Yesterday, you were having minimal conversations, and most of them were about you. Today we had a little back-and-forth, and you had the energy to extend your thoughts over a prolonged period about some of the stuff that I'm working through.

You are improving. I know that you're frustrated because it isn't going as quickly as you want it to, but it is happening, and to my eyes it is happening remarkably quickly.

Trust in the process.

You have my unconditional love and support. Be well, Carla.

3/12/12 - West Virginia, Mountain Mama, Take Me Home

I had something completely different planned for tonight, and then I checked my Facebook feed.

As you know, I am Facebook friends with every single Chris Sypolt on Facebook. There are seven of us. More men have walked on the moon.

Anyway, one of the most active of the Chris Sypolts lives in West Virginia and is likely a distant relative of mine - Fox's parents were from West Virginia (mountain mama, take me home...When this is over we are so going to the Nite Light and drop like $100 into the jukebox.)

Anyway, he's a right-wing Christian Evangelical wacko, but I haven't blocked him because he seems earnest, and it takes different strokes to move the world.

Today's post was why I'm glad I made that decision:

"Unforgiveness is like drinking poison and waiting for the other person to die."

This might be the most important thing I've read. Ever. Not just because of the message, which is powerful in its own right, and comes at an opportune time, but because it is one more strand in this web that I've increasingly become aware of.

There are no accidents. Every single thing happens for a reason, and miracles are more commonplace than you might imagine - you just have to be open to looking for them.

You have my full love and support - believe in miracles, because they happen every single day.

3/13/12 - Carrying The Couch

As with any endeavor that involves cancer, there are inevitably some setbacks where it is zero steps forward and 3 steps back. This day was one of them.

I know you want to be brave. I know you want to solve this with your will. That is incredibly admirable, and a tremendous Big Hairy Audacious Goal.

Sometimes it is wise to remember an important Foxism: "every so often you need someone to carry the other end of the couch."

Go to UrgentCare. Go to GroupHealth. Use your will to demand an appointment and determine if this is in fact normal, or if they can do something to help you.

Better yet, let your sister do it for you. She is an awesome advocate, and she will not rest until she knows that everything that can be done is being done.

Text Messages: 3/14/12 8:03 PM

Carla: Thanks. It just doesn't feel that was. My insides feel broken and empty. I'm just too tired to sleep now. I keep praying things will turn in the couple of days.

Me: Our bodies have evolved to be self-healing. It will recover. Never forget that you are a highly evolved stupendous badass.

3/14/12 - Don't Peek. Seriously.

I wasn't sure what I wanted to talk about today, and then I came across this (best viewed on iPad). Read it before you come back to the email.

http://deadspin.com/5893117/the-shocking-proof-that-tim-tebow-and-tebowing-are-cosmically-linked

Seriously, peeking ahead is strictly frowned upon. If you decided to skip ahead, go back and read the article.

Stuff like this is what convinces me that there is a higher power at work, and that fills me with happiness. I don't know if this means that I should believe in Jesus, or Buddha, or Allah, or Yahweh (in the Latin alphabet it is spelled with an I, which is important to know if you're ever in a situation where you're searching for the Holy Grail, but I digress).

What I do know is that we each have a purpose, and yours hasn't been fulfilled yet. You've touched a tremendous number of lives, but you can touch so many more. Your message is important - I've seen in person how good you are at what you do.

There are a huge number of companies who, if they knew what you do, would be begging for you to inject your humanistic, yet completely company-protecting, style.

You're not going to just survive, you're going to thrive. I know that this is difficult to believe at this moment, but I know this on a level that is difficult to express in words. Keep the faith, Carla. You can do this. Rely on your inner stupendous badass.

Text Messages: 3/15/12 9:45 AM

Carla: I'm very very scared that something is wrong.

Me: It is hard not to be scared of the unknown. You've done a fantastic job to this point, and they will be able to help you, I'm sure.

Me: OK. Try to rest. Believe that you've done the right things all along. Believe that this is Herman saying one last goodbye, because he is such an asshole.

Carla: I don't anymore Chris. I feel like I'm moving in the wrong direction.

Me: I am sending every good thought that I can your way.

Carla: Please do. I need all good thoughts.

Me: Nothing but the best for you.

3/15/12 - No subject line comes into my head at this moment

(There were a couple of more setbacks and challenges with anemia and the burns that resulted from radiation. Carla got a lot sicker.)

It is about 11:00 on Thursday as I'm writing this, and your sister has been kind enough to keep me in the loop about where you stand right now.

First, though, I want to apologize to you for failing you. I took my role as motivator-in-chief too much to heart and as a result missed some signs that I probably should have seen - maybe you would have been able to catch this earlier and things wouldn't have gotten as far as they did. I'm truly and deeply sorry. I should have listened more closely.

In the time since I got the message from Stu, via your sister, about today's diagnosis, I've done some googling and discovered that while this is kind of scary, they are also treatable. The anemia is the primary cause of the weakness that you've felt and the confusion - not chemo brain.

Hopefully one good thing will come out of this - your medical team will pay a bit more attention to you, and we have all learned to speak up when something seems off. You have an incredible force of nature in your corner - your sister is your greatest advocate. Please let her exercise some of that to help.

In addition, they hopefully took a long time explaining all of the side effects and what to watch for. If they didn't, tell your sister. She won't rest until they give her everything that she needs to help you.

I also feel compelled to tell you that The Naturopath got an email from me last night updating him on my perception of how you were doing. Part of it was fueled by the alarm bells that I didn't pay enough attention to, part of it was because I thought you'd be seeing him today and I wanted to give him as much info as I could - while he is extraordinarily perceptive, he hasn't known you for 14 years, and in a case like this I felt like doing whatever I could to tilt the odds in your favor, despite the fact that you probably didn't want me to, was the right choice.

As a result, you can expect a call from him sometime on Friday. I swore him to secrecy on the fact that I had contacted him, but that particular veil has now been pierced. Feel free to let him know that I emailed him, or don't. That's your call.

I'm really sorry that I failed you, and for any suffering that my failure is linked to, but it will never happen again.

You are my most special friend, and I love you more than anything. You're going to get through this, and we are all here to help you. We will do whatever it takes to help you not just survive, but to thrive.

Text Messages: 3/16/12 5:53 PM

Carla: Hey might there be one night a week that you might be able to spend the night?

Me: I can do 7 nights a week. Tell me where to be and I'll be there.

Carla: That should work great but let me confirm the details. This is a different role now that we are not talking about shuffling me to the doctor. This is about more nurse type things so it is not as fun. Just want to be sure you know what you're in for and if you still want to do it.

Me: Unconditional love means there are no conditions. Anything you need, I will be there.

Carla: Okay then. You r now Wednesday man! Bring your pjs and BJ.

Me: Amber is available to handle BJ most nights if 3 dogs are too much. You've got a lot of teammates that you're not even aware of.

Carla: That's great. Tell her thanks.

Me: I will. The awesome part is that she volunteered before I had a chance to ask - like I said, lots of teammates for you.

Carla: I'm so looking forward to you having a day to spend the night and be my nurse! I'm kicking everyone else out for you on Wednesdays!

Me: You've kicked Herman's ass. I can't describe how proud I am of you.

Me: The last week sucked ass for you. No denying that. But together we will put that in our rearview mirror.

3/16/12 - The Natural. Again.

It is amazing, once you get into it, just how much this movie has to offer. It is all out there in plain sight, just waiting to be picked, like a ripe red apple of Truth and Wisdom.

Roy Hobbs: That day in Chicago. Why did you stand up?

Iris Gaines: Because I didn't want to see you fail.

Do you remember the scene I'm referring to - the one in Chicago?

Hobbs has been in a hitting slump for a couple of weeks. Ninth inning, 2 outs, a man on first, down by one. Hobbs drags himself and his slump to the batter's box.

Strikes one and two follow in quick succession. Iris, his high school girlfriend, stands up, her white hat shimmering in the late afternoon sun. There is a commotion in the stands with people yelling for her to sit down. She refuses.

Hobbs looks up, sees her in the stands, and you can see in his body language that he has returned to the state of mind that he had when he was a teenager, when he could do anything he wanted to on a baseball field.

Relaxed, finally, he drills the next pitch into the clock at Wrigley Field. Cue some of the most amazing inspirational music ever.

The situations aren't perfectly analogous, but they are close enough. We, and by we I mean a large number of people - myself, your sister, Stu, your friends, your mom, Amber, John, everyone in your office, Alice, both of my

138

sisters, random people that I've talked to in bars - we are all standing up because we don't want to see you fail.

Your have two jobs. First, relax and concentrate (As Annie in Bull Durham said, this is the secret to both hitting a baseball and sex) - return to your natural non-anxious state. You'll be better able to wage this war.

At the same time, understand deeply what Fox told me again and again and again - sometimes you need help to carry the other end of the couch. All of us who are standing up, because we don't want to see you fail, are your advocates.

If you have a need, don't hold it inside. Don't ask. Just say.

Just as important, accept our help even when you don't think you need it. Tell us what your body is telling you. We are here as your advocates, to speak for you when you can't, to watch over you.

We have one goal, and that is to see you restored to health. Together, we can make this happen.

You are not going to fail. Those of us who are standing up will not allow it.

3/17/12 - (Insert the theme song from Raiders here)

I've been storing up this little chestnut for a while. Have never even seen Last of the Mohicans, but given some pivotal moments in our past, I thought it appropriate to break it out.

Hawkeye: "No, you submit, do you hear? You be strong, you survive... You stay alive, no matter what occurs! I will find you. No matter how long it takes, no matter how far, I will find you".

The truth is, though, that you don't need saving, Carla. You never have. All of the strength you have ever needed is inside of you. You've proven that over the last 8 weeks.

Your body is healing - you can see it with your own eyes that the burns are receding and the blisters are going away. Believe in yourself like I believe in you.

This will end. It is ending. And you are getting better.

Harkening back to an earlier email -

"It was you."

"No, Carla, it was you."

You have my full love and support. Keep kicking Herman's ass all over the place.

Keep up the skeer. Even when it doesn't matter any more.

3/18/12 - Can't think of a subject or a theme

I was very happy to see you today - I know it doesn't feel like it, but the essence of you, whatever makes Carla Carla, is still there and shining through. I understand that this is hard to believe, or to accept, but I've known you for 14 years now - this has, of course, been incredibly difficult for you, and I see that reflected in your tiredness, but it hasn't changed who you are.

It was also helpful to be able to talk to Stu about what the docs said on Thursday. I think that the Gatorade will be helpful in keeping your system a bit more in balance.

It sounds like your friend will be able to take over on Friday nights, which I think will be helpful on a couple of different fronts. First, you get to see some new people. Just as important, your sister and Stu will get a little break, which will help them to do a better job as your primary caregivers.

It really was heartwarming to see each of these people lining up in support of you - each of them pledging to do whatever it takes to support you. While all of us have our quirks, there was one thing that is clear - we have one focus, and that is to help you as you heal.

Healing is taking place, however slowly - you can see it with the burns. Please trust the process. At the same time, if something isn't right, please tell one of us. We will do anything to try to make it right.

I want you to know that this is going to have an end, and it is going to be positive. If it wasn't, your medical team would have already performed the surgery. You're going to get through this. This darkness will lift soon.

You have all of our love and support.

3/19/12 - The Future

Really looking forward to Wednesday night - I know that this is about helping you, but I feel like a fraud when I think about the amount of caregiving time I've been able to provide.

Do not take that as anything more than I wish that I could have done more to help you. Someday we will sit down and watch Casablanca from end to end and this statement will make sense. For now, understand that I am here for you, no matter what you need or ask for. Except for my liver. I really need that.

Digging back into Cryptonomicon again. This is a conversation between a guy who would go on to be a founder of the National Security Agency and one of his main guys, who just wants to finish the war and teach math at a college in eastern Washington. It seems appropriate.

"Sounds delightful, Waterhouse, it really does. Oh, there's all kind of fantasies that sound great to us, sitting here on the outskirts of what used to be Manila, breathing gasoline fumes and swatting mosquitoes. I've heard a hundred guys - mostly enlisted men - rhapsodize about mowing the lawn. But when they get back home, will they want to mow the lawn?"

"No."

"Right. They only talk like that because mowing the lawn sounds great when you're sitting in a foxhole picking lice off your nuts."

I don't want to belabor the point, because you've already figured it out. Sometimes thinking about getting back to a normal, but mundane, part of everyday life is all you need.

So think about what your equivalent to mowing the lawn is. Maybe it is fighting with Earl. Maybe it is arguing with me about politics. Maybe it is cuddling with the dogs, or enjoying a well-deserved cocktail on the deck on a summer afternoon. Focus on normal.

Because that's your future.

Text Messages: 3/20/12 6:45 PM

Me: Are you scared that this will never end, or that it is going to fail?

Me: I can tell you that it isn't going to fail. You kicked Herman's ass all over the place, and soon the surgeons will do their job, and this will be over.

Carla: I feel overwhelmed by all of it.

3/20/12 - It Is Not Too Far

Your text today really threw me for a loop, and I went into full-blown overprotective Galahad mode. That's not necessarily a bad thing. Every so often it is nice to have someone watching over you. I'm convinced that Fox still is for me. And I am now doing that for you.

I want you to know that I am doing that for you now, and that I am at most 15 minutes away - Delores (the Volvo, I'll let you figure out how I got to that name) is really, really fast, and I have a low tolerance for artificially imposed government edicts like speed limits, especially on a seismically suspect structure like the Viaduct, where no cops can hide. But that is another rant, for another day.

I do want you to know that that it is ok to be a little scared. This is perfectly normal. You're facing something awful. Actually, change that to past tense - you've faced something awful. You're now recovering from it. Ever so slowly, but you are recovering.

It is time to dig deep into the Gospel of The Swayze, from Point Break:

Bohdi: Fear causes hesitation, and hesitation will cause your worst fears to come true.

Do not hesitate, even when it seems like it would be easier. This whole experience sucks ass, but you will survive it. Keep kicking Herman's ass. You have come so far, and done so much.

It is not too far.

You have all of my love and support, and if you need anything, all you have to do is say it - it will be provided.

3/21/12 - You Only Thought You Were Getting Out Of An E-Mail

I found out that St. Bonaventure was the patron saint of bowel problems, and got Carla a St. Bonaventure medal, even though as a Lutheran I don't think she was as steeped in the veneration of saints as us Catholics are. I've been doing a little research on St. Bonaventure, and by doing research I mean reading his Wikipedia profile.

This stood out:

"In philosophy Bonaventure presents a marked contrast to his contemporaries, Roger Bacon and Thomas Aquinas. While these may be taken as representing, respectively, physical science yet in its infancy, and Aristotelian scholasticism in its most perfect form, he represents the mystical and Platonizing mode of speculation...

...To him, the purely intellectual element, though never absent, is of inferior interest when compared with the living power of the affections of the heart."

I know that I'm reading quite a bit into this, but on the surface this sounds like either right brain vs. left brain or, more generally, the work-life balance question. After 14 years, I know that these are interests of yours.

He may really be your guy, and not just because of his association with bowel disorders. Something to think about as you move forward.

You're on the path. Keep doing it - soon your house will again be filled with music and good friends and deep philosophical conversations about Bohdi's cryptic statements.

I can't wait.

You have all of my love and support. Don't ask - tell us what you need and it will be provided.

3/22/12 - Today's Foxism

"The second time you get kicked in the head by a mule is not a learning experience".

Ok. We've learned to expect the unexpected. We've learned that your primary caregiver is actually you, and that no two cases are the same.

We've also learned that something new is something that needs to be paid attention to. I'm not trying to be alarmist here, just acknowledging reality - new things need to be examined.

We are all making this up as we go along, just like Harold and the Purple Crayon. I don't want to sound trite, but the warnings in the subway in NYC seem to be applicable - if you see something, say something.

I'm not going to quote from Cryptonomicon again, but one of my favorite characters says the same thing repeatedly: "show some adaptability". You've done that. Continue doing that. Herman's undoing is that he does not adapt. You are smarter and faster than he is.

Keep evolving.

Ok. I am going to quote from Cryptonomicon.

"The Americans have invented a totally new bombing tactic in the middle of a war and implemented it flawlessly. His mind staggers like a drunk in the aisle of a careening train. They saw that they were wrong, they admitted their mistake, they came up with a new idea. The new idea was accepted and embraced up the chain of command. Now they are using it to kill their enemies.

"No warrior with any concept of honor would have been so craven. So flexible. What a loss of face it must have been for the officers who trained their men to bomb from high altitudes. What has become of these men? They must have all killed themselves, or perhaps been thrown into prison."

Remain flexible. This is what you do naturally anyway - I've learned it from you, in part. Keep thinking differently, and keep bombing Herman back to the stone age, no matter what tactics you need to employ.

You have all of my love and support.

3/23/12 - Every Single Minute

Something you said the other day on the way to The Naturopath's office has resonated with me.

You were talking about what you were going to do for your sister and yourself after this is over, and you said that a spa day was inadequate. A spa month, you opined, might be a start.

Here's the thing, and as my brain is swimming in scotch right now, I'll keep it simple. Life is what happens when you're waiting for the big moments to happen. I've spent the last three years getting this out of my system - every one of the Maui trips were things that I scheduled out over the horizon, so I could look forward to them as a reward for myself.

It seemed logical, at the time. But once I had been there several times, I realized that it really was just another place.

More importantly, I finally figured out something I said about 4 or 5 paragraphs ago - life is what happens when you're waiting for a big event. Every single minute of every single day is important.

Be well, Carla. You have all of my love and support.

3/24/12 - The Best Offense

There is a long-held belief in the NFL, and in the US Military, that the best offense is a good defense. Under normal circumstances, this actually works out. Having strong defenses in peacetime usually precludes the need for strong offensive capabilities - your enemies can't bear the cost of attacking.

And then Pearl Harbor and 9/11 happened. Our enemies found that all it takes to cause chaos is to find a small weakness and exploit it. It is funny how we applaud that behavior in Star Wars (the Death Star exhaust port) and are appalled by the practical application of this approach in the real world.

You can look at the post-Pearl Harbor and post-9/11 eras as being essentially equivalent. A weakness was found and exploited. The US, oriented more towards defense than offense, takes a while to get in gear, but once they do kick into offensive mode, they unleash forces that were only dreamed of before.

This is you right now. You have a choice - play defense and hope no more weaknesses are found, or go on the offense.

Yoda was right. Do, or do not. There is no try. Eat. Walk around. Change yourself from someone who is not going to lose (at which you've done very well) into someone who knows they're going to win.

All it takes is one step to start the process. We can all be there to steady you, but you have to take that step and allow us to support you.

It turns out that if you want to win a war, the best offense is not a good defense. The best offense is a good to great offense - if you're advancing, defense rarely comes into play.

You have all of my love and support.

3/25/12 - The Sound Barrier

Loved today's phone call. You're not all the way back, but you're getting there.

In order to make sure I'm not repeating myself, I often check back on the previous week's emails. I tend to take my tone from our conversations, our text messages, and occasional conversations with my spy in your house. That tone shows up clearly in the emails.

Most importantly, if you were to look back a week ago, you would see a much darker theme. That has changed in the last several days.

Here is the bottom line - you are healing. This war has become mental and emotional, rather than physical. And this is a war that you were built to win.

Physical resources are finite. You may have a lot of them, but there is a limit. You have not approached that limit yet. Emotional and mental resources are limitless - they are bounded only by your imagination.

You've been tapping into the mental side for a while, and logic would say that you're reaching a limit. You're not.

It isn't you that bends. You can bend the spoon, no matter how impossible it may seem.

Keep bending the spoons, Carla. This is who you are. You were built for this - you are approaching an exponential curve where all of the tiny steps that you've made will coalesce.

I have often described the first two years at OLM in terms of the "breaking the sound barrier" scene in The Right Stuff. As Yeager approaches the speed of sound, things start rattling around in the cockpit, and the ride becomes a little rough.

Once he gets through the sound barrier, the ride is smooth, and he describes the plane as "climbing like a homesick angel".

Your ride will be that smooth in the very near future.

I really need to watch that movie again. There are so many amazing lines and/or metaphors.

You have all of my love and support.

3/25/12 - Letter to Family / Friends

An update is in order.

The anemia is more or less under control. The burns are healing. We had a scare this week with a very aggressive rash that tested as a staph infection but is more likely a combination of drug interaction and the body detoxifying itself of the chemo drugs via sweating. She's on antibiotics just in case.

The rash was scary not because of the physical effects, but in her words "I've done everything right, and now this?" This is the most clear-cut case of two steps forward and one step back that I've ever seen, and she reeled for a couple of days.

There have been several surgical consults scheduled, so we are waiting on the results from that.

The biggest problem is that she isn't eating a lot, which is contributing to a low energy level. We are switching tactics on her - instead of asking her what she wants to eat, we're providing her with any number of finger foods for snacking rather than larger meals. This is basically Gammy's imperative of "eat, eat" writ large.

Will keep you up to date as events warrant.

3/26/12 - The Finishing Kick

You've gotten through phase one with the chemo and the radiation. You've more or less gotten through the burns, and I am at least partially convinced that some of the rash is caused by your body detoxing through your skin.

Remember, there are only 3 ways out for toxins - poop (still the funniest word in the English language), pee, and sweat. There may be a drug allergy involved, but since you've been taking the drugs all along, mostly, I'm leaning towards the fact that your body is detoxing. It wants to heal as much as you want it to heal.

I was watching you out of the corner of my eye tonight as we were watching TV - you're not itching nearly as much as you were a couple of days ago. This is progress. This is you getting healthier.

You've beaten chemo.

You've beaten radiation.

You're beating this rash.

You're beating the feeling of overwhelming fatigue.

In short, you are beating Herman. You are kicking his ass all over the place.

There is nothing that has been put in front of you that you haven't beaten. You've proven to the world just how tough you are. You're not just a survivor - you are a conqueror.

You are a stupendous badass. You were already one by birthright. You are now one by virtue of your battle scars.

There's just one thing left to do - in running terms, they call it the finishing kick - the ability to pour it on at the end. I know that you don't think you have it in you, but you do, because it is the easiest thing in the world to do.

You need to eat like it is your job.

Lots of small meals - handfuls of almonds and slices of pears and apples all day. Have something close by to snack on. I don't care what tactics you use, but your body needs energy and nutrients to win this war. Give it the means, and it will provide the results.

There is one other thing that I want you to do - I want you to know how proud I am of you. You have done something great. You need to embrace that - YOU DID THIS.

Now let's blow this battle station and go home.

You have all of my love and support.

3/27/12 - An Alternate Hypothesis

Switching to purely tactical matters here for a moment, I've done some research into psoriasis and have developed an alternate hypothesis that this is actually a good sign.

While scientists are unclear about the causes of psoriasis, they have classified it as an autoimmune disease, by which they mean one where the body's immune systems start to attack its own cells, in your case newly formed skin cells.

On its face, this doesn't sound great, but think about the implications for a little bit.

Your immune system is so strong that in addition to kicking the ever-loving crap out of Herman, your white blood cells have decided that during their off hours they're going to start hazing the skin cells that have been generated in the wake of the radiation burns.

Our bodies and our immune systems have evolved over millions of years - your white blood cells have a certain capacity for prioritizing problems, and the fact that this is happening now suggests a real reason for optimism, because newly-created skin cells are way down the priority list for attack.

In addition, the fact that your immune system is on such a hair-trigger alert status, and is capable of responding in such force, is a good sign as well.

I want you to think about these things and to realize that you are in fact rebounding, no matter how you feel physically. I'm not going to trivialize what you've done by comparing it to me going to the gym, but the analogy is apt - I always feel the weakest after I finish a workout, and then a day or so later, as my body recovers, I feel a leap forward in strength and energy.

You haven't had a day off in a very long time. As a result, the good feelings that would normally occur haven't shown themselves. And yet you've continued to get stronger.

Two weeks ago, you weren't really up to being able to put butter on a piece of bread (I'm exaggerating, just go with it), but as of yesterday, you were making your own lunch.

Progress is happening, whether you believe it or not. It is apparent to those of us who are around you, even though you may not be feeling or seeing it.

Trust in the process, and trust your body. You are a stupendous badass by birthright, and I am infinitely proud of you.

You have all of my love and support. Keep kicking Herman's ass.

3/28/12 - The Watershed Line, Part II

I'll keep this short, mainly because right now, after what I saw tonight, I'm convinced that you are on the right path.

I wish that for a moment you could step outside yourself and see you as I do and then compare it to two weeks ago. As scared and as emotional as you were, I was just as scared and emotional. But everything has changed since then.

I can only imagine what you have had to endure. But that part is in your past. It will always be a part of you, but it is receding and it can't hurt you any more.

Day by day you are getting stronger. I see it every time I visit. Take comfort in the fact that you are awake more than you are asleep, that you eat tacos instead of veggie shakes, that you're helping to clean up after dinner rather than falling asleep in the middle of a conversation.

You are healing. There is no doubt about this fact. Be patient and let your body do its work. It is doing its job.

You have all of my love and support.

3/29/12 - Keep Up The Skeer (Lost Track Of How Many Times I've Used This As A Subject, Let's Call It 10)

Let's move back in time, oh, about 8 weeks or so.

You: "This is going to be the hardest thing I'll ever do."

You were, of course (and, as usual), right. This has been so insanely difficult for you that I can't imagine (and in truth I don't want to imagine) what it took to get through it.

But you have done it. You've done everything that was asked of you and more. You have nothing left to prove on the toughness scale. Maybe the hiker/mountain climbing guy that had to cut off his own arm could give you a run, but I'd bet on you - you've outlasted him.

We are coming up on 3 months of you living with this. You've displayed strength, toughness, and most importantly, adaptability on almost every single day.

Herman never had a fucking chance.

Keep doing what you're doing - now that you see that it is working (the rash is receding, you're eating a bit more easily, amongst other things). Now that you have had a taste of winning, refuse to give ground.

You have all of my love and support.

Text Messages: 3/30/12 4:48 PM

Me: It's all coming together.

Carla: I hope so. Tired today and a bit restless. That is not good for me.

Me: My plan was to win Mega Millions and provide you with a nurse that looked like Antonio Banderas. Sad to report that this won't be happening.

Carla: Shattered dreams. Oh well thanks for the thought and somehow I will get by.

Me: I'll settle for you kicking Herman's ass to infinity and beyond.

3/30/12 - One More Step

About a million years ago, I spent a winter learning to run in preparation for the Beat the Bridge run.

I had really never been a runner before I started on this trip. This was back when I was still living near Greenlake.

One day, I went down to Greenlake and started to run. The verb run here is charitable. I kind of stumbled forward in a way that was faster than walking, if only barely. I think I made it 300 yards before quitting.

The next day, I had one goal - get past what I had done the previous day. I lasted 310 yards. It took about 2 months, but eventually I made it all the way around the lake - 2.8 miles. I really can't describe the elation that came with accomplishing this goal.

I know you're asking the question - "why is he telling me about something that happened 10 years ago?"

Here's why - because the incremental approach still works. Because getting past what you've done before is an incentive.

If you are up and moving under your own power, start to write these things down. When you wake in the morning, know what you did yesterday and resolve to take one more step.

That one step is important. It asks you to push a little further, I know. But your body is built to deal with this. It will respond.

Keep taking one more step.

Be well, and sleep well.

3/31/12 - Pop Quiz, Hotshot

Let's return to something that I sent to you at the height of the storm.

Iris Gaines: There's the life you learn with, and there is the life you live after that.

For a short period of time, Fox was a high school teacher. He talked at length, though, about how easy it was to spot those students who were Aware. In my time at OLM, I've seen the same thing - we've been fortunate in that our screening process has eliminated a lot of people that did not display Awareness. Well, except for She Who Shall Not Be Named. We are not perfect.

You, my friend, are awash in Awareness. If I ever am dumb enough to start another company, you're going to be employee #1, because you really get it on a very deep level, and people like you are incredibly few and far between.

I could continue on this set of masturbatory paragraphs at great length, but all it would do is bore and embarrass you. You've already figured that part out.

I go back to something I asked a couple of months ago - this experience has, I think, freed you of an internal filter - basically, your tolerance for bullshit has dropped below zero.

Pop quiz, hotshot - what do you do? Do you continue to play the political game, exchanging small wins and smaller losses, or do you stand up and proclaim that the Emperor is buck-ass naked?

You don't have to do this, of course. You can keep fighting with Earl and the rest of the people in your office, and take the wins where you can find them. This can be a very good life.

There is a difference between a good life and a fulfilling life, though. A fulfilling life goes beyond what is expected. You have that trait in you. You know it. I know it. You don't accept good enough.

I don't know what you're going to do with the life you live after the life you've learned with, but I can't wait to see the results.

Be great, Carla. Be well. You have all of my love and support.

3/31/12 - Letter to Family / Friends

It looks like the worst is probably over. Carla is up and moving around on a reasonably regular basis, and she is eating like a 15 year old boy - basically, if we put it on a plate, it will be gone 10 minutes later. The rash she has been experiencing cleared up almost overnight. As far as her recovery goes, we are approaching the elbow in the exponential curve.

I made soft tacos on Wednesday and spaghetti on Thursday - she demolished both of them and suffered no ill effects, unlike in previous weeks where eating anything induced awful cramps. If anything was going to be a problem, it would have been my recipe for 5-alarm spaghetti, the chief ingredient of which is enough garlic to hold off a battalion of vampires.

There is a surgical consult on Tuesday, where I'm hoping that they finally show her that what she's gone through has some meaning, and that Herman has withered up or is not even there any more.

At this point, emotionally and mentally, she's about 85% of the way back, so I'm concentrating on trying to engage that last 15% - this is the part that really makes Carla Carla. Hard to describe it until you've seen it in person.

Thank you all for all of the support and good thoughts. You can't imagine how they have helped.

April

4/1/12 - Inhaling Bliss

Today's meditation is from the book about introverts that I was talking about earlier. This is in the context of a class/seminar on addressing a fear of public speaking:

"Take it slow. There are only a few people out there who can completely overcome their fears, and they all live in Tibet."

Just a really great set of sentences that really put our lives into perspective. Fox put it another way - the only perfect person ever was executed like a common criminal. Being human means having to deal with anxiety on an almost daily basis.

I want you to know that as far as I can tell, you're doing everything that can be done, and you've been doing it since day one. I think you should tell your medical team that you are still really tired, mainly so that they know where you are.

You're quickly coming to the last phase of this ordeal. Based on our conversations, I have the feeling that you're thinking a lot about Tuesday. That is completely ok. It is also ok to have a lot of emotions and/or anxiety and/or unsettled feelings. That's what the quote above is all about.

This is the time when the part about inhaling bliss and exhaling attachment really comes into play - it has application when dealing with pain, as you've discovered, but where it really is valuable is in managing your emotions and anxieties.

I've seen it work. I've felt its power and calming influence. It can work for you, and I encourage you to lean on it.

One other thing - as I said at the beginning of this, you have had to actually do this by yourself, but you've never been alone. The number of people who are doing their part to help you really is staggering. You can do this, because you have all of their love and support.

Be well. Be great.

(Tuesday was a reference to a meeting with the surgeons who would tell her how much of her colon they needed to take out and whether her colostomy bag was going to be temporary or permanent. One of the reasons that she started with chemo and radiation, rather than surgery, was because she was terrified that she would have to live with a colostomy bag for the rest of her life. It was one thing that she just didn't think she could live with.)

4/2/12 - Day One

You may recall that on the day you started your treatment, I titled the email Day One. Today is your next Day One. The chemo and radiation part are in your past. You drew the line in the sand and declared that Herman would progress no further. Since then you've been napalming his ass into oblivion.

Today you hopefully see the results of your efforts, and they'll finally show you what you've accomplished. More importantly, you'll see the path to the end of this. It has to have been incredibly difficult to do this without any feedback, but you have ground it out, day after day after day. I can't describe how proud I am of you.

I quote myself, from the first paragraph of the first of these emails, way back on January 30th:

"You can do this. It won't be easy, but you can do this. You have it in you to overcome it. I've seen it in you."

Think about what you've overcome since then. Think about the heights you've scaled. You are absolutely unbreakable, and once you get past this next phase (which I have absolutely no doubts that you will), the world opens up.

Morpheus in The Matrix: ...There's a difference between knowing the path, and walking the path.

You have walked the path, Carla. Your body has endured repeated insults to deliver you from Herman / evil / dark forces. But your mind, the thing that makes you you, is still more or less the same. A bit older, a bit wiser, of course, but the spark in you has not been diminished.

I've said this before, but there have been moments during this where your essence has filled the room, when you've become more than you ever could imagine you could be. These moments have been hard to describe, let alone capture, but I've seen it. You're a special person.

All that is left to do is to walk the final part of the path, which is way easier than the path that you've walked so far. You can do this.

Be great, Carla. Be well.

Text Messages: 4/3/12 8:47 AM

Carla: Your last two emails have been exceptionally inspiring. Thank you for continuing to send these. They mean a lot to me,

Me: Thanks. I've kind of hit a nice groove recently. Keep up the good work!

Me: Good morning! Wanted to let you know I was thinking of you and wishing you good luck today.

Me: The one thing I want you to remember is not to be intimidated because they are doctors and you aren't.

4/3/12 - Quo Vadimus

I'll explain the Latin later.

I didn't hear from anyone about how the visit to the surgeons went today, so I am going to assume the worst, that they can't save enough tissue and will have to perform a permanent colostomy. If this is the case, I am so sorry.

At the same time, I want you to know that you did everything right, everything you could do. You didn't leave anything out on the field.

This isn't the outcome that you wanted, but it is an outcome that you can live with. More importantly, it means that your long-term prospects are actually better, according to what I've read - they won't take any chances and will take out any tissue that even has the potential to be a problem. You won't have to live with this hanging over your head. It will be a part of your past.

I've heard and read a lot of anecdotal stories about people who are living full and happy lives after this procedure - my neighbor has an uncle who was waterskiing with one in Arizona as recently as last week. I know it is hard to believe, but he has had the option of reversing the surgery for the last 6 months and has chosen not to, as it really doesn't affect his ability to go about his daily life.

All of these things, of course, are easy to say when you're not the one who has to do them. But I know you. You have displayed your toughness throughout this ordeal.

Let's stop and get semantic for a minute. In the metals world, strength is the ability of a material to withstand an applied stress without failure. Toughness is a measure that requires a balance between strength and ductility (ability to be stretched).

Drago was high in strength. Rocky was high in toughness. There is a difference.

When you didn't think you could handle the chemo, you did.

When you didn't think you could handle the radiation, you did.

When you didn't think you could handle the burning or the cramps or the rash, you did.

I just checked my Time Since app - by my calculations, at 3 am on Wednesday, you will cross over 2,000 hours since this started. Finally you are at a point where you can see an end, and while it isn't everything you hoped and prayed for, what I know is that my best friend will still be here for a long time to kick my ass when I do something criminally stupid, and for that I am eternally grateful.

You have every right to be deeply upset by this. You have every right to be deeply upset by a lot of things that have happened in the last 3 months. But this is coming to an end. There is a clear path out of the wilderness.

You are deeply loved by a lot of people, and this will not change those emotions even an iota. At the end of the day, that's a pretty good way to go through life.

You have all of my love and support.

Be well, Carla. Be great.

4/4/12 - Simplicity

(Based on my knowledge of Carla and many of the things she was thinking, I instinctively knew that she was having a hard time coming to terms with her upcoming surgery and the aftermath. Losing something as fundamental to the human experience as the ability to use the restroom without relying on an external bag is not a simple transition.)

I've been debating with myself for the last 24 hours about what to say tonight.

You know what? I still don't have an answer, and I'm operating on assumptions and suppositions and inductive reasoning, none of which help me to know what to do to help support you.

But none of that matters, really. What I want you to know is that you are loved, unconditionally, and we will do anything that you need to help you.

The person that you are has not changed in the last 48 hours.

That's it. It is that simple.

Be well, Carla. Be great. I'll see you tomorrow afternoon.

4/5/12 - Do.

I've talked about an awful lot of things during the last couple of months. I know that at some level they helped you in some way. Most of them have been full of rhetorical flourishes, and they were written with a specific purpose in mind - to keep you motivated and moving forward.

Tonight, we're going in a different direction, at least for one email. Tonight I'm going to talk about me, and if there is one thing I ever am able to get through to you, it is to beg you not to become me, or at least don't become me from roughly 2001-2009.

To use a phrase from the past, I am only going to tell you this once.

I am not telling you this story for any other reason other than that you're at a point where you can choose how you want to live your life. My story is not comparable to yours when it comes to the suffering you've endured. That's not what it is about. What this is about is the Life You Lead After and the choices that you make. In order to put things into context, I have to tell the whole story.

In short, don't make the mistakes I've made.

You know most of this story, at least in bits and pieces. This is the first, and likely the last, time that I will ever lay it out in one place. I do it not to inspire sympathy, or even to inspire you, but rather in the hopes that you don't make the same mistakes that I did.

The beginning was relatively innocuous. I had a fever over 103 for 3 or 4 days, and my neck started swelling. Finally I made an appointment with my doc, where he drew some blood and poked his finger in my ass.

8 hours later, after the blood work was done, they called me to tell me that my blood sugar was 700 and that I needed to go to the hospital immediately. The ER pumped 2 bags of fluids into me. They took more blood and x-rays. The X-ray nurse, a fetching Latina lass, complimented me on my nipple ring and exhibited a look that 3 hours later I finally defined as "smoldering". Pity that I never followed up.

At 3 am the doc finally came in, after I had been there for 5 or 6 hours, and told me that I was diabetic, then walked out. The sum total of my discharge instructions was that I should drink clear fluids and call my doc for follow up. I really hate doctors.

I spent the rest of the night alternately shivering and pouring out sweat. I went through 3 sets of sheets in 4 hours. Just for fun, my neck swelled up to about 2 times its normal size.

At no point in my life, even through Catholic grade and high school, have I ever said that many Hail Marys at one time. Finally, dawn broke.

I saw my doc the next morning, after the longest 4 hours of my life. I remember the conversation.

Him: "So, you're diabetic"

Me: "That's what they said."

Him: "Do you want to know how it happened?"

Me: "Does it fucking matter?"

In the years since, I've devoted an excessive amount of time trying to come up with a slightly less profane, yet equally as witty, reply, usually involving intense questioning, sometimes involving waterboarding, as to whether the doc owns a DeLorean and a Flux Capacitor, and possibly a Mr. Fusion.

I have an active imagination.

The next day, on a referral from the doc who was clearly hiding his access to a time machine, I went up to Pill Hill to see an endocrinologist who was supposed to take over my diabetes care. She was a dream come true - from New Zealand, which was close enough to Australia that I asked if she knew Olivia Newton-John. She was not amused.

I spent most of the appointment imagining her in black spandex and leather and singing Hopelessly Devoted to You, until my world exploded again with her announcement that the Doc with the DeLorean was wrong - instead of type II, which you get because you're fat (I was), and can be treated with a pill, I was type I, which means insulin injections. Every. Single. Day. For the rest of your life, every time you eat.

She then introduced me to a fucking cunt who had no feelings, I mean nurse, (I often get these terms confused), who showed me how to use my blood glucose monitor by holding down my hand and jabbing something shaped roughly like a tack halfway through my index finger in order to collect a small blood sample to run through the machine.

It was only in later years that I was to learn that opening a vein was not required to accurately judge sugar levels. This would have been helpful information at the time.

The docs up on Pill Hill subsequently referred me to the Joslin Diabetes Center for instruction on how to inject myself, because patient care is apparently best when you outsource it to a non-profit.

After 3 visits to Joslin, the nurse handed me a syringe and said it was time to do a dry run. I looked at it. Time stopped. I could hear the beating of my heart and the flow of blood through my arteries. I told her that the first time I needed to do it by myself.

I felt ashamed. I felt weak. I felt terrified. I was not ready to give my life over to this. To have it rule my destiny. This was not me. She gave me a syringe and told me to try it over the weekend.

I put the syringe on the coffee table next to a bottle of 12 year old scotch. On Sunday, I got really drunk and attempted to inject myself. The only problem was that instead of doing that, I dropped the syringe and bent the pointy part.

(Patience, young Jedi. I am working my way around to a point eventually).

I went back and got another syringe. This time I had only enough for a buzz, not a full-on drunken episode. It was time for the injection. What a letdown - I never even felt it going in. No pinch. No feeling like I was being split open.

Here's where we finally circle around to the important part.

I have continued to have an adversarial relationship with every doc that has been involved with my case, except for The Naturopath. I spent 9 years hating the world for doing this to me.

This came out in my relationship with my docs, who I viewed as adversaries to be outwitted, and in the long line of women who I rejected because I was an asshole and wanted the perfect situation to present itself.

I hated the world and everyone in it. This is no way to go through life.

I threw away 10 years of my life because I was mad at fate. It took my experience with one girlfriend, and the aftermath, where I was as close to eating my gun as I could have been without actually doing it, to realize one single truth.

Life isn't worth having unless you are willing to spend it on something other than anger and regret.

I know that this has taken too long, and that the payoff wasn't that earth-shattering. I just don't want to see you make the mistakes that I did.

You have an army to support and love you. Reach out to them whenever you need to.

Sleep well. Be well. Be great.

4/6/12 - Transitions

The Universe, it would seem, is imbued with a certain sense of irony. You and I have been swimming in Change ever since I have known you.

I know for a fact that I have a hard time understanding how, when I show people a new and better way of doing things, even when it makes their life easier, that they resist and don't want to make the change. I have to assume that you've experienced the same thing.

Yes, I'll grant you the point that what is about to happen is not necessarily an improvement. It is, of course, something that needs to happen so that you can put all of this behind you, and to the extent that you'll be able to eat without pain, it is better than the current state.

But it is still a massive change, and change is hard on everyone, even for those of us who believe ourselves to be Change Agents. I think adverse change is actually harder on people like us - we're used to making the changes, not having the changes made to us.

I think that's why I reacted so badly, and against my own interests, when I was diagnosed with Type I, and why I continued to do so for years. This was something that was completely out of my control, something random that was being imposed on me.

It took a long time for me to come to terms with that, and the fact that it took such a long time is really my own fault. I look at who I was when it happened, and I don't even recognize myself. I look at who I was right before I came to terms with it, only 3 years or so ago, and I still don't recognize myself.

You at least have the advantage on my experience in 3 specific areas. First, you're far more self-aware than I was. Of course, this is not a high bar, as my dog BJ is more self-aware than I was. Still, you're way more in touch with who you are, and you process things at a higher level than I was capable of.

Second, you have been operating on a far higher spiritual plane than I do for as long as I've known you. That's a huge leg up - you're open to seeing the world in a way that I am only now starting to understand.

Finally, The Naturopath. I think you know what I am talking about. He is the West Coast Distributor of the philosophy of removing attachment from our lives. Attachment can cause so much pain - you've seen it happen to me, and the stuff that he does is geared to easing that pain.

Transitions take time. You probably remember the old Archie Bunker routine where Edith is going through change of life and Archie is yelling at her that she has 5 minutes to change. You can't force a transition - it has to happen on its own timetable.

What I'm saying is that it is perfectly OK to take time and to feel as you process this change and come to terms with it. Rushing it will only lead to long-term damage, as I talked about last night.

Everyone is aware, at some level, of all the breathing exercises that women in labor go through. What you're doing right now is its spiritual/mental equivalent.

What I'm trying to tell you, a bit ham-handedly, is that you have all of the tools that you need to face this and to manage the transition. You know the psychology way better than I ever will. You understand the spiritual dimension. You've got your own personal Yoda in The Naturopath to tie it all together. And you've got people like your sister and Stu and myself to listen to you.

What good would I be if I didn't try to bring in at least one Yoda quote per week?

Yoda: No more training do you require. Already know you that which you need.

Luke: Then I am a Jedi.

Yoda: (shakes his head) Ohhh. Not yet. One thing remains: Vader. You must confront Vader. Then, only then, a Jedi will you be. And confront him you will.

I'd love to tell you that you don't have to face Vader, but you do. You are already a Jedi. You already know that which you need.

Be well, Carla. Be great. Trust in yourself and the fact that you are loved unconditionally by more than you know.

4/6/12 - Letter to Family / Friends

It has been a while, so time for an update.

Carla continues to recover - the psoriasis outbreak that got her so upset last week is pretty much gone. There are one or two spots left, but they are shrinking.

The big ongoing problem, if we could call it that, is how tired she is. I'm trying to figure out whether or not to make more of a concerted effort to get her up and out of bed in order to kick her system into gear.

This week's big news is that surgery is scheduled for April 17. Although she was able to reduce the tumor substantially, the docs have told her that in order to make sure she is cured, and not just in remission, is to take out everything. The meaning of this is that she will have a permanent colostomy bag - once this procedure is performed, it cannot be reversed.

She has made the very difficult decision to go this route because they've told her that it is the only way to be really certain and to put this in her rearview mirror.

That's not to say that she's handling it well. This is a major step for anyone to take - as much as the bodily function that will be replaced is kind of gross, the permanence of this fact is weighing on her. Also, there is the embarrassment factor to cope with.

Took her to see The Naturopath on Thursday and he was able to get her calmed down as to the mechanics of how the bag works. She had been operating on totally faulty assumptions, which contributed to her highly emotional state.

So now we wait. She's able to eat more easily and has the appetite of a teenaged boy right now, and she's spending a lot of time processing this change and trying to come to some level of acceptance.

She has an appointment with The Naturopath the night before the surgery for some heavy-duty acupuncture and massage to help get her anxiety levels down, and I continue to send her an email each night. As of this morning I'm over 28,000 words and am considering using Amazon to publish them as an e-book. We'll see what comes of that.

Thanks to all for the support.

4/7/12 - I'll keep this short

While our experiences are not exactly analogous, I can tell you this - we have more in common than you might expect, and I'm a pretty good listener. We won't find all of the answers, to be sure, but maybe I can help you find a little peace.

I'm here to listen to you, to help support you, and I can do it as someone who has had many of the same feelings and thoughts.

All you have to do is pick up the phone or send a text - just ask and I can help you carry this couch.

You have all of my love and support.

4/8/12 - Juice

I will freely admit that this goes a bit off the beaten path, but there have been too many weird coincidences recently for me to discount it.

I have been aware of a phenomenon for the past couple of years where I will get a very strong, repeating image of some piece of pop culture arcana over a couple of days. The feeling, for some reason, initially started with specific scenes from episodes of MASH. I would visualize the episode for a couple of days, and then, when I was looking around for something to watch, I would happen upon that specific episode (there were 251 of them, so this is a .04% chance), almost always down to the scene that I had been thinking about.

There is a 99% chance I've already lost you at this point, but I assure you that this has happened to me at least 25 times. The pattern is almost always the same. In the past 18 months it has expanded to other scenes from other pop culture stuff that I'm way too familiar with. I have been able, with about 75% accuracy, to predict movies that will be showing on the usual cable channels on Saturday afternoons.

Yes. I know that this sounds insane. For me, it is evidence that the Universe is weird. This is likely the least useful psychic power of all time.

This came to a head for me about 3 days in advance of us watching Zack and Miri Make A Porno - I kept having flashes of the scene where the drunk guy interrupts the filming of one of the scenes. When it happened on-screen I was convinced that something odd was happening.

All last week I was thinking of two scenes - one from 40 Year Old Virgin (when Elizabeth Banks is in the hot tub), and one from The Girl Next Door.

Obviously, the 40 Year Old Virgin has come and gone on Saturday night. Really awful pun there. But I keep coming back to the other movie, The Girl Next Door, which I can't find anywhere in the upcoming showings list on IMDB. This is unusual for me - once I lock onto something this strongly, it usually happens quickly.

Here's the scene I keep flashing to. I'm including the entire IMDB quote, without clipping the things that don't apply.

Matthew: "Moral fiber. So, what is moral fiber? It's funny, I used to think it was always telling the truth, doing good deeds, basically [mumbling] being a fucking boy scout. But lately I've been seeing it differently. Now I think moral fiber's about finding that one thing you really care about. That one special thing that means more to you than anything else in the world. And when you find her, you fight for her. You risk it all, you put her in front of everything, your future, your life, all of it. And maybe the stuff you do to help her isn't so clean. You know what? It doesn't matter. Because in your heart you know, that the juice is worth the squeeze. That's what moral fiber's all about.

Let's set all of that insanely long text aside for a moment and concentrate on one salient question:

"Is the juice worth the squeeze?"

Only you can answer this question. I know what my answer was when it was put to me. I ran and hid like a 5 year old. It was too far. There is nothing wrong with running and hiding. The only problem is that the question remains, and it is a question that will wait for an answer.

It took some time before I understood that the juice was worth the squeeze.

I can tell you from my experience that getting from the bombshell to living your life takes some time. There is no way to rush it. You know what I am taking about.

What I can tell you is that the juice is worth it, regardless of the squeeze. Life is awesome.

I'm here. Stu and your sister and a cast of hundreds are here. We want to listen to you, we want to help support you no matter what you want to talk about.

I keep coming back to one thing. Unconditional love. My religion teachers spent a lot of time talking about this back in high school, but I've only started to understand it recently. We are here for you, to listen, protect, and serve. There is nothing that you can ask that we won't try to deliver.

To that extent, and to the point that I don't have anyone watching over me (I really miss Fox), the juice is absolutely worth the squeeze.

You have all of my love and support. Sleep well and be great, Carla.

4/9/12 - Waterworld II

I'm really glad that last night's message was helpful. I was cringing a little bit when I sent it - I know that it makes me sound like a crazy person, but I assure you that it is 100% true.

I talked at the end about unconditional love, but I don't think that I did it in the right context - yesterday I was talking about how those of us who are around you will take care of you no matter what the circumstances.

What I really wanted to talk about, and didn't, was a basic, simple idea. No matter what happens to you physically, the unconditional love remains exactly that. We look at you the same today as we looked at you 3 years ago, and we will look at you in 3 months, and in 3 years.

I've learned the hard way that there are two kinds of people in the world - those who have earned the right to have their opinion affect me, and everyone else. For those in the latter group, I listen politely sometimes (most of the time not so politely) and then go on my way.

For those in the former group, I listen politely and then go on my way. There is only one person who has my happiness as their only goal. Me.

I go back to something that I talked about early on - our conversation at the Rocksport, where you kind of blew me away with your statement that you admired how I went through life. Coming from you, it was really high praise.

The funny thing is that I've kind of used you as a role model for years - you have always marched to your own drummer, and in times of uncertainty, I haven't necessarily gone the What Would Carla Do route, but I

188

have seen how you acted in similar situations, and I have taken my cue from that.

I want to bring in something from the 13th Generation book by Neil Howe and Bill Strauss, where they attempt to describe the best traits of our generation - "if you have a job that needs to be done, and you're not particular about how the job is done (in many cases, you don't want to know), then these are the people you want to talk to."

You and I are those people. Without putting too fine a point on it, while we may not be whole physically, we can solve problems that others throw their hands up at. We are fixers.

Look at what you did when your office flooded so badly that I asked when Kevin Costner planned on filming Waterworld II there. You took it in, and then settled down and started solving problems. The office was back up and running within days, and it wouldn't have happened without you there to make it happen.

Do you really think that after next Tuesday you would be less able to solve that problem, or one like it, again? No. Of course you don't.

I've kind of drifted around tonight. I know that. There's just so much I wish that I could communicate to you, but I know that it is something you have to experience at your own pace.

If there is only one thing that I want you to remember, it is that no matter what happens to your physical self, it cannot touch your mind or your heart. You alone decide who Carla is. You were pretty fucking good before this started. Nothing has happened to change that.

You have all of my love and support. Be well, sleep well. Be great, Carla.

4/10/12 - Cosmic Tumblers

We haven't talked in a while, so I'm not sure where you are emotionally. This isn't a criticism, just a recognition of facts. I'm looking forward to hanging out with you on Wednesday and Thursday night.

I don't want to make assumptions, so I'll talk about me for a little bit.

I want you to know how thankful I am that you allowed me to be a part of this. The times I have come over and made dinner, or have just been there, have been some of the most fulfilling points in my life. I tried to explain it, and failed, so let me be direct - this is the first time since I started at OLM where I knew without a doubt that I was in the exact right place at the exact right time.

"There comes a time, when all the cosmic tumblers have clicked into place, and the universe opens up to show you what is possible."

- Ray Kinsella, quoting Terrence Mann, Field of Dreams.

I've had those moments, for which I am forever grateful. But these emails aren't supposed to be about me. They are supposed to be about you.

I really hope that you can understand what I was talking about last night - that a change in your physical makeup does not affect who you are. It does take some time to process this, but I can guarantee that it will happen, and that in a very short time you will look back at your fears and be able to say, truthfully, that you are done with them.

You have all of my love and support. Sleep well and be great.

4/11/12 - Steel

I want to talk to you for a moment about change. Not about the physical change that is coming soon. I want to talk about the change that has come over you since this started.

I go back again and again to our conversation that we had outside your bedroom on the weekend before treatment began. You told me that this would be the hardest thing you've ever done, and it has more than lived up to that particular billing.

You have been tormented in ways that I just can't imagine. In the end, unfortunately, it wasn't enough to overcome how much Herman had grown undetected. You fought a great fight. You deserve a better outcome.

But what I really wanted to talk to you about tonight was what I heard in your voice, compared to what I heard at the end of January. There is only one word to describe it: Resolve.

There was steel in your voice tonight. This was the voice of someone who has been to the absolute limits, and who has refused to give in. I know that you're worried about the surgery itself, but what I heard tonight is something really simple that I can only sum up in a variation of a Richard Dreyfuss quote that we've used over the years:

"You want to be a cancer survivor? Then BE a cancer survivor."

You're going to win the war, Carla. You have shown all of us what it means to be Unbreakable.

Sleep well, Carla. Be well. Be great.

4/11/12 - Letter to Family / Friends

With surgery on Tuesday, she's not allowed to eat anything after Saturday, so we are doing kind of a potluck buffet - bring your favorite dish and let her sample a little of each thing.

While I am good at only a few things, the thing I always felt I was best at was waffles and homemade maple syrup. On top of that, the waffles freeze really well and are easy to reheat in a toaster for quick meals.

For obvious reasons, I haven't had that in 11 years or so, and my memory of the recipe is lost to history.

Any chance that any of you still have a copy of the recipe?

4/12/12 - The Other End Of The Couch

I've talked about this several other times, but one of my dad's favorite sayings was this - "sometimes you need someone to carry the other end of the couch."

As you approach the end of your fight, I think it is natural to try to retreat within yourself. Millions of years of evolution have taught us to separate from the pack to lick our wounds and, if necessary, to distract the attention of predators away from the main group. Evolution hasn't yet caught up to humankind's social dynamic yet.

This is unfortunate, in that our genetic programming denies us the thing that studies have shown again and again to be a key to surviving and thriving. In other words, somebody else to help carry the couch.

Rely on us - we have each been here for you through each step of the way, and we're not going to abandon you now. You are loved and supported by more than you will ever know.

Sleep well, Carla. Be well. Be great.

PS - really looking forward to surprising and delighting you on Saturday.

4/13/12 - Everything

I can only imagine this, but knowing you, I'm going to guess that you've spent a lot of time worrying about Tuesday and everything after. Given what's going to happen, I think it is natural to worry about things that are out of your control.

The thing is, though, this is in your control. You could have said that you wanted to do another round of chemo instead of surgery, but after hearing everything the docs had to say, it was ultimately your decision based on the fact that this is the way to ensure that this is over.

I've said all along that it takes courage to do what you've done. You're displaying it yet again by taking this step, because there is only one thing that matters.

I've done a little research on the surgery, and everything that I've read is that you're basically the ideal candidate - your youth, the fact that you've been able to keep your weight up, and the fact that Group Health does a lot of these procedures are all things that help to make certain that it is successful.

I know that this won't help a lot with your anxiety levels, but maybe it helps a little.

In the past, I've sent you some stuff written by Drew Magary. He usually posts articles full of dick jokes at Deadspin.com. He recently recounted, however, the story of the birth of his son, who was born 7 weeks premature. The final paragraph says everything:

"He's in the NICU now. They put him in a special incubator, and he'll have to stay there for a few weeks, but that's OK, because they gave me a wristband, and wristbands make me feel 80 percent cooler. I can waltz right past the suckers in the waiting room and go into the kickass sick-baby unit. I'm shocked CBS doesn't have a shitty hourlong drama called NICU on the air right now. I stole a swaddling blanket from his incubator and now I sleep with it every night because it smells like him. He's breathing, and he's eating, and he's peeing, and he's pooping, and everything will be all right, even if it isn't all right. Alive is what matters. Alive is everything."

If you're interested, this is easily the best thing I've ever read from him, and probably the best thing I've read from anybody in at least a year.

Sleep well Carla. Be well. Be great.

http://www.deadspin.com/5900973/pain-is-a-gift-and-other-notes-from-a-terrified-father-during-a-seven+week-premature-birth

(Of note, but of very little value to the story, is that Drew Magary is one of my favorite writers, and I've been deeply influenced by his style and his ability to use f-bombs effectively. If you are not put off by a writer who makes jokes about farting, I highly recommend any of his now-prodigious amount of output).

Text Messages: 4/14/12 5:21 PM

Carla: Thank you for coming over and participating in my pre surgery feast!

Me: It was my pleasure. Thanks for swallowing my terrible waffles. They do get better.

Carla: Nonsense they were like dessert. And the bacon was wonderful. Thank you.

Me: I love you unconditionally. No matter what happens, I will be there for you.

Me: With poorly made waffles and correctly made bacon.

Carla: Okay not that I'm vain, but I noticed that no one told me I looked good today. It's catching up to me isn't it. Be honest.

Me: No. You do look good. The key thing I've looked for is your moments of strength.

Me: Hearing you tell stories about your friends today is all I need to know about how you're doing. Through all of this, your Carla-ness shines through.

Carla: Thanks.

4/14/12 - Resilience

As you get closer to the end of this phase, I want you to look back, not to relive the pain, but to think about what you went through, and to realize one simple truth:

There is nothing that can conquer you.

You've been battered, to be sure, but you're still here. You're still standing.

Today was a reminder of how things used to be - a house full of friends and music. It reminded me, as Terrence Mann said in Field of Dreams, of all that once was great, but more importantly, it reminded me of what can be great again. It reminded me of what you've been fighting for all along.

We're going to have a lot of afternoons like this in the coming months, and for you they will be even sweeter knowing what you had to do to enjoy them. Thank you for showing me what it takes, and what is important in life.

Be well, Carla. Be great.

4/15/12 - Unleashing

It is amazing to me how the old stuff keeps coming back again and again. This is from Fast Company in 1999:

"Freedom is actually a bigger game than power. Power is about what you can control. Freedom is about what you can unleash." - Harriet Rubin

I know you're focused on getting through the next hour, the next day, the next week. But after this experience, after all you have gone through, I am really looking forward to see what you are going to unleash.

The question is this - if you lived in a world without rules, without social restrictions, with no constraints on the decisions you make, what would you make the world into?

After all that you have endured, isn't it time to start seeing the world differently?

I love and support you. See you around 3 pm or so.

4/16/12 - Thank You

My plan for today was to give you this note in the form of a card that you could open in the morning. Since I won't be coming over to pick you up for The Naturopath, I guess I have to switch to plan B in order to get it into your hands, and since I don't know how much you'll be checking your phone in the AM, I'm sending it now in hopes that you'll read it before you go in for surgery.

Thank you for letting me be a part of your life.

Thank you for all of the amazing conversations we've had.

Thank you for kicking my ass when it needed to be done.

Thank you for forgiving me when I did things that were unforgivable.

Thank you for listening when no one else would.

Thank you for inspiring me to be great when good enough was an option.

Thank you for staying true to who you are in the face of something so difficult that I can't even imagine it.

Knowing you has been the best thing that has ever happened to me.

Thank you for being my friend.

May the Lord keep you in His hand and never close His fist too tight.

Be well. Be great.

4/17/12 - Letter to Family / Friends

I'll know more when I visit tomorrow, but it looks like we are out of the woods.

Text Messages: 4/18/12 8:14 PM

Carla: Slowly starting to feel better. This will take some time.

Me: Yes. You are on the path to health. I really can't tell you how happy I am that you are going to be OK.

Carla: Today was a better day. I took a walk and ate some solid food. The doctors were pleased. Hopefully getting better everyday.

4/19/12 - All Good Things...

I don't even know where to start, Carla.

I am overwhelmed by a sense of relief so strong that it envelops me in its embrace. Seeing you tonight, seeing the life in your eyes and in your face and your Carla-ness just shining through was powerful.

It isn't nearly enough to make up for what I've watched you endure over the past 3 months. But what it is is a fresh start. The past no longer has power over you. It can't hurt you any more.

You're still with us, and for that I am profoundly grateful. You're almost done with the most difficult thing you will ever do. There are still some steps to take, and you're going to be changed by this. I hope that you focus more on the gift of cancer than on the curse.

And with you now out of danger, and on the road to recovery, I think that it is time to bring these emails to a close for a while. You no longer need them to survive. You no longer need them to help you get through the night.

You're not going to get rid of me that easily, though. You can still expect a 2,000 word rant to show up in your inbox from time to time. I think, though, that I was fortunate enough to learn some stuff from you. That the limits of what we can endure are way beyond what we ever think we can. Most important, though, is learning to separate the really crucial stuff from the ebb and flow of life.

Thank you for teaching me that. Thank you for allowing me to call you my friend.

Be well, Carla. Be great. Be who you are.

4/19/12 - Letter to Family / Friends

Just spent an hour with her. You wouldn't believe the change. She looks great. She's alert and funny and...well, she's Carla.

They expect that she will be back home by the end of the weekend, as she has shown great progress.

Text Messages: 4/20/12 8:52 PM

Carla: Things are coming together but it was good that you left when you did. Major colon blow. Stu handled the whole thing like he was on Grey's Anatomy!! Amazing.

Me: You know what's amazing? Your attitude.

Me: I've always known how strong you are. You can stop showing off - it makes us mere mortals feel inadequate :) (That is the first and last emoticon I will ever use).

Text Messages: 4/22/12 9:49 AM

Me: Checking in to see how you're doing today.

Carla: Much better. Almost like starting over but today is a much better day. Thanks.

Me: You will be able to do this, Carla. Do it at your own pace - you know yourself better than anyone.

Carla: I am so fucking over all of this. I can't even put it into words.

Me: I know. It is almost over.

Carla: No it's not. It's not almost over that's the problem. This doesn't end.

Me: Please trust me when I say I know how that feels. It does get better. I wouldn't be standing here if I didn't.

Carla: I know but my heart and soul just feel beat to hell

Me: That's because they have been. But you're still here. You're alive. Alive is awesome. Your heart and your head will recover like your body is doing right now.

Text Messages: 4/24/12 10:09 PM

Carla: Tomorrow is too soon. This is a hard transition and my pathology did not come back as expected so I am in no mood for visitors or conversation. I hope you feel I have adequately thanked you for everything you did for me during this time and if not let me say thank you so much again.

Me: Carla, you don't need to thank me at all. I appreciate that you want to, and I happily accept your thanks.

Me: I love you unconditionally. If you need anything, please let me know.

4/27/12 - Letter to Family / Friends

Apologize for the lack of updates. The situation has been unstable. I also apologize for doing this via email, but speaking seems not to be something I can do right now.

During surgery, they found fluid in her abdomen. It has been tested and found to have cancerous cells, meaning that her organs have effectively been bathing in whatever this stuff is.

Her prognosis is now 1-1/2 to 2 years with chemo, or considerably less without.

May

5/6/12 - Letter to Family / Friends

There has been some more bad news.

I could provide the technical term, but that would just lead to a lot of Googling and unnecessary discomfort on your side. This is a negative development for Carla, and it appears that she has moved into Stage IV (as opposed to Stage III).

There is a chance that chemo could hold it back for a while, or the often-prayed for miracle, but I'm not particularly optimistic, having spent way too much time Googling the technical name. The outcomes associated with this problem give her a very small chance for any kind of survival beyond several months.

I'm working with The Naturopath to try to bring her some peace, but at the end of the day there is no way to describe this entire experience other than that it sucks.

Seeing your best friend at 123 pounds, unless she is a workout freak, is jarring. This sucks a lot.

5/11/12 - Letter to Family / Friends

We have both good and bad info today. I'll start with the bad, as it was scary when we heard it, and became less scary later on. I'm also holding off on the good news because I like happy endings.

The bad - she has developed a couple of abscesses in her abdomen. On some level, this could be expected; she was so backed up that it was impossible to clean all the stool out, which is apparently what led to the abscesses. She's back in the hospital for a couple of days of high doses of antibiotics and possibly surgery if she doesn't respond.

How is this possibly going to lead to good news? Well, on its face it isn't. However, the fact that her body has healed enough from the first surgery that they would even consider a second is a great indicator of how much she has healed. She is getting better.

Here's where things start to turn up. The Naturopath was making a house call when the phone call announcing her tests arrived. He is, as I've noted many times, seemingly the only medical professional involved in this entire saga who recognizes that there is an entire patient behind the symptoms.

Had the call come in when he wasn't there, she would have quickly slipped into yet another wave of crying and assuming that she wouldn't leave the hospital if she went in. That didn't happen. He was able to actually talk to the other doctor and explain things to Carla in a comprehensive way that kept her out of the spiral.

He ended up staying about an hour and a half, and as he had taken the bus down, I gave him a ride back to his office afterwards. More on that later.

Some decisions were made - they have been able to move up the appointment with one of the oncologists to next week, rather than the week after.

In addition, they are flying to Phoenix next Saturday to be evaluated at Cancer Treatment Centers of America, which claims to have a higher percentage of favorable outcomes in late stage cancers than is the norm. The Naturopath endorsed that wholeheartedly - he even was in school with a couple of the naturopaths there. CTC apparently specializes in a whole patient concept, healing the mind, body, and spirit, so that when you meet with your medical team, it is an actual team. This fits well with Carla's outlook.

Even better, should she go that route, her insurance covers her 100%.

Ok - the conversation with The Naturopath in the car. He said she is healing really well and that her lab results look great. She's lost a lot of weight (down to 119), but that is normal because she hasn't been eating, which is also normal. He deals with a lot of cancer patients and said that after this type of surgery it is not unusual for the appetite to come back slowly, and he expected it would be back very soon.

He also said that now that he's seen all the lab results and been actually able to evaluate her in person that this is all a minor blip. He's been treating cancer patients for about a decade, so I'm going to defer to his expertise and not the fear and anxiety that I've been channeling for the past 3 weeks, as well as my excellent Googling skills.

But he went further. Let me use his exact words: "I'd be very surprised if we all (including her) didn't look back in a few years and have a laugh about how scared we were in light of something so minor."

Maybe this is me grasping at straws, but he went even further: "I had to have The Conversation with another patient today. I was prepared to do it again with Carla. I see no reason to have that conversation with her anytime soon."

He said, when we were at the house, that when he sees a cancer that doesn't make sense - in this case, no family history, no risk factors, way younger than typical, he recommends getting three opinions, and often times the three will vary wildly.

By the end of next weekend, we will have 3 opinions and will be able to see a way forward. And that's the best news I've had all month.

Text Messages: 5/13/12 8:52 PM

Carla: I will be here another day at least. We are not done yet. More tubes to be placed, etc. I am starting to lose it depression wise. I know I'm anxious but I'm starting to feel full on depressed. I need to get through today's procedures even though they are hard.

Me: You're going to be ok, Carla. If you're feeling like that, please make sure that your nurses know and call the Naturopath. He can help you without even touching you.

Text Messages: 5/14/12 7:54 PM

Carla: Things went well today. Feeling less anxious trying to relax a bit. Thanks for listening yesterday. Another dr appt tomorrow and Thursday. I'll keep u posted.

Me: I'm very happy to hear this. You can do this, Carla.

5/19/12 - Belief Levels

It was so nice to talk to you this evening. It was so nice to hear that through everything you've endured, you're still with us. I don't mean physically - I mean that the Carla I know is still here. Because that Carla can prevail against any odds.

I saw enough of the hospital routine to know that they asked you every time that they saw you about your pain level on a scale of 1 to 10. They didn't ask you about your Belief level.

I think that this it is just as important to track your belief level, whether it is with me, or Stu or your sister, or whoever you designate to keep track of these things. Pick somebody, and make sure that you report this level to them on a regular basis, and you let them know that you want them to ask you about it.

Empower them to pass this info along to The Naturopath - I can get you his direct email address if you decide to route this info through someone else.

Be honest about how you feel - we may not be able to react immediately, but I think that it is fair to say that your support team will do what we can, outside of direct support from The Naturopath, to help you to keep the Belief and to help you see a way forward and through.

I have no idea if what you are attempting is even possible. The Naturopath says it is, and that is all I need to know. I know, innately, that the only way that you're going to be able to do it is if you Believe you can. And doing it means putting one foot in front of the other.

For now, this means beating the infections, as well as whatever other steps that The Naturopath gave you. That's the only task to worry about right now.

You can do this, Carla. Go and do it. It is not too far.

Text Messages: 5/20/12 1:35 PM

Me: Hope you're still up at around a 9 on the belief scale. Keep healing.

Carla: Im okay. Bach to the hospital again today. Same ol thing.

Me: Good to hear. Keep healing.

Carla: Trying my best.

Me: Your best IS good enough. You can get better if you believe you can.

5/20/12 - Letter to Family / Friends

Just realized that it has been a week or so since the last update. Not a lot of news at this point. (Ok, just realized how long this email ended up being - there may be a nugget or two of new info).

Carla spent last weekend in the hospital, as planned, getting a high dose of IV antibiotics, and left Sunday with a drainage tube and IV bags full of antibiotics still attached to her. Emotionally, this was not a high point in this saga - it felt to her like one more case of one step forward and two back.

The place in Phoenix has said that they can't even see her until these infections are cleared up, which is not for another week or two. In the meantime, she and Stu saw a highly rated oncologist here in town on Tuesday, and they're still trying to get callbacks from a couple of others locally.

The gist of the conversation with the oncologist was this - "we're really at the limits of what can be done. Our experience is that you're looking at 12-24 months. About the only good news is that once you get past this infection, you won't really experience a lot of pain."

So it comes down to, from the oncologist's perspective, 3 choices: 1) do nothing, and she'll last one to four months. 2) Go with aggressive chemotherapy, which will get her closer to the 24 month window but will leave her sicker than she has ever been (having watched her for 4-1/2 months, that is an insanely high bar). 3) Go with a milder chemotherapy that will likely mean that she's looking at a 12-18 month window.

She has resigned from her job and applied for Social Security Disability benefits. These are the bad times.

I stayed the night with her on Thursday. The IV for the antibiotics is somewhere near her lower back (she wasn't volunteering to show it to me, and I really didn't want to see), which makes it uncomfortable for her to sleep, and the colostomy bag is on her lower left abdomen, meaning that it is almost impossible to get comfortable. Might as well throw sleep deprivation into the mix.

At any rate, she and I only had a couple of brief conversations on Thursday night, but it is fair to say that the operative word was despair. We watched a couple of episodes of Veronica Mars that I had purchased for her (a highly underrated show - if you're looking for something to watch, I highly recommend it), and she fell asleep more or less in mid-sentence.

I've been keeping The Naturopath up to speed with all of this, and he made a house call (a house call? What is this, 1940?) on Friday. I don't know the specifics of the conversation, but Carla and I talked for a brief time yesterday.

When I visited Carla in the hospital, I was struck by the fact that anytime a nurse came in, she was asked what her pain level was - this was their way of monitoring how she was doing. What they really should have been monitoring, at least from my perspective, was her Belief level - at this stage of things, The Naturopath told me last week, the only people who recover are the ones who Believe that they can.

So when I talked to her on Saturday, I asked her what her Belief level was on Thursday, and what it was after The Naturopath visit. The Thursday answer was "like maybe 2". The Saturday answer was a definitive "9". The Naturopath is amazing for his ability to give someone real hope.

As I told him in an email I sent on Thursday night, after she had fallen asleep -

"My sense of her tells me that she has gotten this far on guts and survival instinct. She can take the pain and discomfort (she's been stronger than I ever expected her to be in that area). As I said, this is the first time I've ever witnessed something like this, but in talking to her it sounds like her (reverting to 7th grade Dungeons and Dragons mode) Belief and Hope attributes need some assistance."

I don't know what the next steps are. I know that I feel a lot better than I did on Thursday, and I know that the Carla I talked to on Saturday sounded more like herself than at almost any time since January. If Belief is a prerequisite for beating this, she has it.

Finally, things veered into the Realm of the Weird with a text message late Saturday from my ex, who was responsible for connecting The Naturopath and I. Like most of my exes (Carla included), I've maintained some level of correspondence, and I've kept her up to speed on the Carla Saga.

Anyway, she had a dream on Friday night where she and I visited Carla. Kelly described the house with surprising clarity, especially since she's never been there, and met Carla for a total of maybe 3 hours at the end of 2009. The substance of the dream is that she found herself brushing Carla's hair and promising that she would make a full recovery.

Like I said, we're out on the far end of the bell curve. This has been a year of firsts, but I've seen a lot of things during this process that makes me think that there are no coincidences, that there is something larger at work. That is enough to give me hope.

I apologize for sending such a long email and thank you all for reading it - I've found that writing is a better outlet for me than curling up in a ball and trying to determine exactly how much fluid I can push through my tear ducts (the answer is a surprisingly large volume).

5/21/12 - My Favorite Things

This is obviously a work in progress. But we will write it together. In the meantime, here is the original to inspire you:

Raindrops on roses and whiskers on kittens
Bright copper kettles and warm woolen mittens
Brown paper packages tied up with strings
These are a few of my favorite things

Cream colored ponies and crisp apple strudels
Doorbells and sleigh bells and schnitzel with noodles
Wild geese that fly with the moon on their wings
These are a few of my favorite things

Girls in white dresses with blue satin sashes
Snowflakes that stay on my nose and eyelashes
Silver white winters that melt into springs
These are a few of my favorite things

When the dog bites
When the bee stings
When I'm feeling sad
I simply remember my favorite things
And then I don't feel so bad

You can do this, Carla. The way through is paved with Belief.

5/26/12 - I have a message for you

This has been building in me for some time. The Naturopath kind of lit the match a couple of weeks ago when I drove him back to his office and he told me that what you are going through is a bump in the road, and nothing more.

I struggled with understanding that but trusted his judgment. And ever since then something has been brewing in me. I haven't been able to put a finger on it, as I've tried to come to grips with what you are going through and how I felt about it.

Finally, this afternoon, I was able to figure out what The Naturopath had sensed, even from the first visit to him that we made:

You're not done yet. You have a larger purpose that God or the Universe or whatever put you here for. You have to get better in order to fulfill that purpose - I have no idea what that purpose is, but you have too unique of a set of skills and talents and abilities to offer to this world.

This is why I've been sending you these texts about believing lately, and I'm finally putting a name to why I've been doing it. You have a larger purpose to fulfill. It lies at the intersection of your joys and the world's (for lack of a better word) needs.

Find that purpose. Actively search for it. Believe.

I love you very much and I am looking forward to seeing you on Monday afternoon.

5/28/12 - Advice from my cousin John

(With the bad news still fresh, Carla decided that if her time was limited, she wasn't going to spend it confined to her bedroom. She and Stu decided to buy a RV and go out on the road to see America. At first I hated this, especially the fact that she would be away when and if something bad happened, but her reaction, and the reaction of other friends was basically "Fuck Yeah! Do that!" I came around to that line of thinking fairly quickly.)

I have been keeping selected family members updated on what's going on.

One of those is my cousin John, who graduated from Harvard with an MD and spent the last 10 years accumulating more degrees in his field of infectious diseases. He seems to be fairly competent and an impartial adviser, although actually graduating doesn't seem to be a high priority.

He has been incredibly helpful to me as I've tried to interpret medical jargon. Here is his response to my latest update. I trust him completely and offer his thoughts to both of you completely uncensored. Okay, not completely uncensored. He had a typo in the third paragraph that I fixed. I am who I am.

"Unfortunately, what she's experiencing with the abscesses and fistula isn't uncommon. I battle this sort of process regularly.

"I completely understand how she's approaching her decision-making at this point. Getting additional opinions is certainly reasonable, and she should be comfortable being up-front with physicians when they make their recommendations. They won't know that she has these sorts of plans for a trip and such, unless they ask (which they won't) or she offers (which she should).

"It's her life and her body, and she needs to do what she feels is best for herself. Her decisions may factor in her family and friends, but shouldn't need to defend it against a physician's push for further treatments, etc.

"Should she undertake any trip, she needs to discuss the plan with a physician who's going to help her through it.

"There would be challenges, but they should be able to manage these hurdles (like making sure she has pain meds if needed, etc.).

"Hopefully, she'll get some additional thoughts and suggestions from the other docs, which may offer some new angles for consideration.

"I absolutely support you both in whatever course you decide to take. Let me know if I can be of any assistance."

5/30/12 - Letter to Family / Friends

There have been, as they say, some developments.

Carla asked me at the last minute to come over this evening, as Stu and his band got an unexpected opportunity to play somewhere in town.

There was a teleconference between Carla, Stu, her second oncologist, and her third oncologist, both of whom work at Group Health. The upshot of that call is this:

- The first order of business will be the removal of all the drainage tubes, as the docs believe that whatever fluids are present will be reabsorbed by the body - there is no reason for her to have to deal with the tubes.

- One of the docs is of the strong belief that whatever is going on (neither Stu nor Carla elaborated), it is very treatable with chemo. It can, in fact, be put into remission.

- She's going to have a port put into her chest on Monday and she'll receive a take-home pack of chemo that will be delivered over the course of 48 hours. This will happen every two weeks. After 4 rounds, they'll check what effect it has had.

- She's been assured that the side effects will be very mild (no pain was, for her, a prerequisite for doing this), and while she may lose her hair, it will grow back. She's ok with that, and I offered her my wide selection of Steelers hats for when she wanted to look stylish.

- Stu actually bought the RV today and they are still planning on going on a bunch of shorter trips over the next several months as the chemo courses play out. She was really animated when she was talking about the places they were going to visit. If, after the first 4 rounds are evaluated, no progress has been made, they'll be saddling up and heading out for 6 months on the road and invited me to join them for long weekends when I can.

This is easily the most un-fun roller coaster ride I've ever been on.

June

6/1/12 - Letter to Family / Friends

What goes up...

Carla got to the hospital on Thursday, excited to have all of the tubes removed and finally be able to have a pain-free existence. Because of the placement of the tubes, particularly the one on her bottom, in combination with the colostomy bag, there is really only one position that she can be in, and it is very uncomfortable. Sitting normally or laying on her back is incredibly painful.

And yet again, her one hopeful moment was taken away when the docs told her that they had made the decision to keep the tubes in for "as long as possible".

Assholes.

Any semblance of hope was crushed by this. It would have been better if they had never said a word about the possibility of taking them out.

I expressed my reaction last night in an email to a friend:

"All the optimism from a couple of days ago is gone, and I feel stupid for even having a little bit of hope that at a minimum she might be comfortable.

"At what point are they going to stop torturing her, not physically, but emotionally? How the hell do I look her in the face and say that she's going to heal when she can't ever seem to catch a break and her docs seem to be actively working to take away hope?"

Chemo starts Tuesday, rather than Monday, although my belief that the docs will actually do what they say they will do has been permanently and irrevocably shattered. Now I'm just waiting for the other shoe to drop, the one where the doc who said this could be put into remission says something like "Oh, you're Carla? I was looking at the chart of someone named Darla. I'd be surprised if you're able to survive the drive home."

And with that sunny thought, I shall now summon the bartender and demand the vast quantities of alcoholic beverages to which, after this week, I feel I am entitled.

(Full credit needs to go to Neal Stephenson's Cryptonomicon for the large majority of that final paragraph.)

Text Messages: 6/2/12 9:05 AM

Carla: I'm getting ready to meet my new class one RV. So excited. Should be here within the next two hours. I went dancing across the USA

Me: Awesome!

Me: You need to name your RV. Maybe have a christening with a bottle of champagne.

Carla: Great idea!!

Carla: I know you think this is crazy but it makes me really happy.

Me: I saw it in your eyes when you were talking about it. I know that it makes you happy, and that's all I care about.

6/2/12 - A little help from the family

From my sister Jenny – a good idea that may help with comfort levels

"Hi. Just thinking this morning and an idea came to me for Carla. Go to a fabric store or craft store. Get a big square of foam. It usually comes in pillow size. Get foam at least two inches deep. Cut out holes where the drainage tubes are. You might need to cut a line to the holes so that you can pull the tube stuff through. You might want to try it with a paper template first so it comes out right.

"Ta-da, you have a comfy pillow for Carla. You will just need to check every once in awhile that it is not causing her red marks on her back. If it is, just change the position of the tubes. Or maybe cut out a canal for the tubes. If you have an electric knife, it cuts foam very easily. We have done stuff similar for the residents at Vincentian House."

6/3/12 - No subject

I've been talking to my friend Michael, who used to be a nurse in Harborview's ER before he and his wife moved to LA. You both may remember him from Solstice a couple of years ago - he was just coming off the night shift. He had some insights that I think you should both be aware of as you contemplate the next steps. He is really blunt, but I appreciate that approach:

"I have found Oncology to be the most inexact area of medicine and have avoided it my whole career as a result. I paraphrase a discussion with an Oncologist - and I have heard this innumerable times before - 'you have cancer. We will do some radiation to burn it out, some chemotherapy to try to kill it, you will get burned, sick, lose your hair, 30% of your body weight, spend every day throwing up. When we are done you might get better. Of course, you might not.'

"Even the best Oncologists have little real insight into treating cancer. In the last 30 years we have cut the mortality rate for heart disease and stroke by 70-80%. The mortality rate from cancer has not changed. 0% improvement in 30 years of smart people trying to figure this shit out. In my opinion, every case is one more experiment they hope to get it right and learn something. This is not any comfort to those in the middle of it unless the MD is honest from the start."

Michael is both smart and compassionate. Take from these paragraphs what you will, but I thought it was important that you heard from someone inside the profession as you are making Really Large Decisions.

Michael has always been a really good guy (despite my low standards for women, I have insanely high standards for guys, and he passes all of them) and I want to give you both as much info as possible as you make decisions. I can put you in touch with him if you want to ask questions directly.

6/8/12 - Letter to Family / Friends

Good news to report, for a change. She started chemo on Tuesday - 4 rounds, 48 hours each, every two weeks. At the same time, they finally took out the tubes, and did it in such a way that she didn't feel a thing (in marked contrast to previous tube-related procedures).

I stayed the night on Thursday. The change was remarkable - she was just completing her second consecutive pain-free day in 6 months. Think about that for a second. Hard to imagine it, and the change in her mood and attitude and outlook was astonishing. She can sit or lay down in any position, and she can sleep through the night.

The chemo leaves her pretty tired, but so far she seems to be tolerating it fairly well. Washington state's liberal attitude toward medical marijuana has eliminated the nausea typically experienced in these cases. I recognize that not everyone on this email list shares this perspective; I've seen the medical benefits in action and my opinions have done a 180 in this area.

The last piece of good news is her weight. She bottomed out at 117 pounds, roughly 55 pounds from where she started. In the last 10 days, she's rebounded and is up to 129.

I remain cautiously optimistic that she will find a way through.

6/15/12 - Letter to Family / Friends

I could post something flowery, but that would be a load
of horseshit. Imagine the second-to-worst case scenario.
It is worse than that. If you really want details, I can
provide them. I can assure you that you don't want
details.

3 rounds and 35 days left. These are the bad times.

I have some insights into the nature of humanity as a
result of a mind-blowing visit to The Naturopath, and
some conversations with Uncle Chuck, and from watching
her struggle, but these insights are not yet fully formed;
I'm still trying to figure things out. I'm still trying to fit
everything in to some sort of a framework that makes
sense.

Yes, Uncle Chad, I know that this is a fool's errand. Humor
me. Spock-like devotion to logic is about all I have left.

For those of you who have a framework for
understanding the world, what is it, and why does it work
for you?

6/24/12 - Letter to Family / Friends

It has been a while since the last update - I've been holding off because I didn't want to jinx things. Then I realized that jinxes don't exist, except for the Pirates, and the way they're playing right now, anything is possible.

The first two rounds of chemo are done - she did not do well with the first one, for a couple of different reasons, mainly due to medical ineptitude. Because of the nature of the approach that they are taking, these rounds are by necessity pretty strong to start off with. It was compounded by the fact that the calculations they used approached her as if she was a 200-pound man.

The results were not good to see. She dropped from about 122 to 112 before it was time for the second round. I took her to see The Naturopath two weeks ago, and she didn't have the strength to a) walk into his office, or b) keep her lips closed. Not good times. Of course, after 90 minutes with The Naturopath she came bouncing out. That dude is seriously amazing.

In addition, they had, prior to the first round, given her an injection of something meant to protect her bone marrow - this had the side effect of bumping her white cell count to stratospheric levels - she maxed out at 28,000. Because one doc wasn't talking to the next doc, the second one looked at the numbers and came to the conclusion that cancer had spread everywhere.

Belying that conclusion, however, was that her cancer marker had only moved from 8 to 10. A large part of that move could be attributed to the ridiculous overdose of chemo juice they had given her.

Between rounds one and two, also, all of the complications that she had been dealing with cleared up,

231

allowing her and her docs to focus only on one thing - the rounds of chemo that remained.

By round two, sanity had started to prevail as doc one and doc two actually decided to talk to each other. They figured out where they had gone wrong and decided to dial back the chemo strength to about 75% of the planned dose, meaning that she should be able to tolerate it better.

The Naturopath, too, was not his usual self in that he hadn't told her specifically to eat normally - she thought she was supposed to be on a raw food organic diet, which contributed to her weight loss.

Now that everything has been straightened out, there is a possible benefit to the fact that she survived the overdose - it was so strong that it likely killed off any remaining cancer cells, and the last three rounds are now just insurance.

When I picked her up for a The Naturopath visit last Thursday, a couple of things had changed - her color was way better, which she attributed to the fact that she was now able to eat and was up to 2,000 calories a day, and as a result her energy levels were way higher. This was being helped by the fact that Stu's parents made the trek up from Arizona and will be staying for 6 weeks to help out. Stu's mom apparently specializes in high-calorie meals, which explains the fact that her husband's beer belly has its own zip code.

She's also been able to get to a good balance with her pot consumption - basically, she's going through about an acre a day (yes, gross exaggeration, but Stu is on a first-name basis with the hippies at the local dispensary), but it both eases the nausea and gives her the munchies, which allows her to eat as if it was her job.

When I dropped her off on Thursday at the house, I saw something that I haven't seen in months - old Carla. She was talking about the fact that The Naturopath had told her to lay off of red meat, and as she was saying that she looked me in the eye and gave me an exaggerated wink that told me that she'd be sending Stu out for a Big Mac later that evening. Cynical/Funny Carla is still around and kicking.

She will, of course, follow the spirit of his request, but her attitude is that she's earned the right to have a hot dog or a couple of slices of meat-lover's pizza without guilt.

One last anecdote - as I was driving her home from The Naturopath visit, we spent a lot of time talking about where we were going to have dinner when the chemo rounds are over in a month or so - she and I had originally planned to have dinner at a local steakhouse for my birthday back in January, but she had to cancel as she felt terrible (3 days before she was diagnosed). The fact that she is planning for the future is significant.

As for me, I went to see The Naturopath for a reboot a couple of weeks ago. I hadn't been there in several months for myself, and to add insult to injury the last time I'd been in the gym was at the end of January. The resultant buildup of negative energy took a real toll on me, which came through in many of the emails. I simply didn't have the energy levels to even contemplate visiting the gym, and the downward spiral perpetuated itself.

After the reboot, I've been to the gym 5 days a week, and there have been zero breakdowns. Part of that is attributable to the recent improvement in prognosis, part of it was due to being able to work off excess energy in the gym. After the initial 10-day adjustment to the change in my physical routine, during which I was basically bathing in Aspercreme (getting old sucks, but is way better than the alternative), I'm basically back on track.

Now that the tale has been told, I want to pass along something that Carla and I have been talking about as a result of her interactions with Western medicine and watching her being turfed from doc to doc, with zero teamwork between them. The Naturopath told her specifically during her last visit that her case has been a classic example of how docs focus on their own narrow specialties and lose any kind of understanding that they are treating a patient, not a disease.

While we rightly hold docs in high regard due to their skills and their training, there is a problem - docs don't go out of their way in explaining everything that is going on and the implications of tests and different events. They assume that their diseases/patients will acquiesce to their greater knowledge. I myself am still waiting for my primary care doc to explain the implications of some test results from 2007.

The doctor may not enjoy it, but everyone has a need to understand everything that is going on with whatever diagnosis they are presented with. I use something I stole from our internal systems improvement process at OLM - whatever the subject, you can generally get to a root cause by asking the question "Why?" 5 times. The point is that accepting information from an authority figure without questioning, especially when it deals with your own health, is a good way to get into trouble.

Thanks for reading the latest epistle, and for the support during the last 6 months.

Text Messages: 6/25/12 6:55 PM

Me: I know you are in the midst of yet another trial. Do not lose faith. There is a long list of people who love you. You can do this.

Me: I love you and have complete faith that you can see your way through. All you have to do is be who you have always been.

Me: No compromises. No retreat. No surrender. Keep up the skeer.

Carla: Thank you. I'm trying my best and hardest to get through this. Each day brings new challenges and new reliefs.

6/26/12 - Alternate fuel sources

I sent a text a while back about a conversation I had with The Naturopath, but I didn't have the time to fully develop the thought.

We were talking about genetic selection, and he dropped this bomb: the brain is the only organ that can run on both glucose (our traditional sugar-based fuel) and ketones (the waste products of respiration).

The only way that this is possible is through evolution, and some insanely difficult famines.

The Naturopath then took it a step further - he has interviewed a large number of Holocaust survivors, always with the same question - how did you get through it?

The unanimous answer is that they were able to tap into a spiritual version of the dual-fuel mechanism that exists in the brain. We all have a life force. It has been bred into all of us, and when we need to switch fuels, we can do it. You're doing it right now, without even realizing it. You have a support system that has been genetically engineered to help you at this exact time. Feel its power. Draw your strength from it.

To quote Yoda in The Empire Strikes Back: "Luminous beings are we, not this crude matter. You must feel the Force around you; here, between you, me, the tree, the rock, everywhere, yes. Even between the land and the ship."

You have a second spiritual fuel source. Tap into it. It is bred into your genes. It is inexhaustible. It will sustain you.

No retreat. No surrender. No compromises. You can do this.

Text Messages: 6/27/12 7:30 AM

Me: I love you unconditionally. I'm not the only one. Keep being the person who overcame her fear of public speaking. Keep being the woman who survived the flood.

Me: Tom Clancy, in some of the later novels, described Jack Ryan as "a good man in a storm." I can't think of a better description for you. Keep following your instincts. AND KEEP KICKING CANCER'S ASS.

Carla: Thanks for sending the inspirational messages again. I've missed them and they really help my spirits. Thank you.

6/27/12 - Baby steps

I was messing around, looking for something to talk to you about tonight, when my completely insane Uncle Chuck decided to weigh in on the question of spirituality:

"I think one of the problems is that Catholic education continued to feed us 'baby food' when we were not babies any more. We were ready for adult food but they kept trying to ram down our throats mashed peas and mashed carrots. We wanted T-bone steaks and baked potatoes. There is a completely different part or subculture of Catholicism that we were never taught or exposed to -- the mystical Catholicism, the intellectual Catholicism: Tolstoy, Merton, Chesterton et al."

I'm still trying to figure out how I feel or manage spirituality - I know that you are way ahead of me on these things, and not just because of what you've gone through for the last 6 months. What have you discovered? What do you draw on? What sustains you?

I miss hanging out with you and will see you this weekend.

I love you more than you will ever know.

Do not give in. Do not accept defeat. Adapt, Improvise, and Overcome. There is a way through, and you can find it.

6/28/12 - Coincidences

From Signs:

"People break down into two groups. When they experience something lucky, group number one sees it as more than luck, more than coincidence. They see it as a sign, evidence, that there is someone up there, watching out for them. Group number two sees it as just pure luck. Just a happy turn of chance.

"I'm sure the people in group number two are looking at those fourteen lights in a very suspicious way. For them, the situation is a fifty-fifty. Could be bad, could be good.

"But deep down, they feel that whatever happens, they're on their own. And that fills them with fear. Yeah, there are those people.

"But there's a whole lot of people in group number one. When they see those fourteen lights, they're looking at a miracle. And deep down, they feel that whatever's going to happen, there will be someone there to help them. And that fills them with hope.

"So what you have to ask yourself is what kind of person are you? Are you the kind that sees signs, that sees miracles? Or do you believe that people just get lucky? Or, look at the question this way: Is it possible that there are no coincidences?"

I think, after 14 years, I know what kind of person you are. I'm pretty sure that I know what kind of person I am, and it has grown stronger as I've watched what you've endured.

I have become more and more convinced that there are no coincidences, that there is a reason for everything. We are not on our own.

Let me repeat that: WE ARE NOT ON OUR OWN. SOMEONE / SOMETHING IS LOOKING OUT FOR US.

You're going to survive. You're going to thrive. I can't explain how I know this, but I know it as surely as I know my name.

The big question is this - there is a life you learn with, and the life you live after that. I posed this question to you back in February; what are you going to do with the life you live after the life you've learned with?

I love you more than you can possibly imagine. Keep being the most Carla that you can be.

No retreat. No compromises. No surrender.

6/29/12 - Let's pick a date

We're going big or we're going home. We're eating lobster and steak and oysters and salmon. Pick your favorite restaurant, and pick a date. Probably not Cutter's, or Icon (where you were asked to leave), or Capitol Grille (the Pan Incident) or El Gaucho (I remember somebody being asked to leave, I just can't remember who).

Pick a date. Pick a restaurant. You and I will be there. Be aggressive and trust in your recovery - don't pick a date in November. Set the bar high. Be the person that I've always known you are.

I love you and know that you are getting better every day. Believe it and it will happen.

6/30/12 - To failure

One of the nice things about having a personal trainer
was that I never had to worry about being crushed by the
bar when I was trying to prove my manhood on the bench
press. The other good thing was that I could get into the
failure zone without fear.

The failure zone is this magical area in weightlifting
where you are really able to build muscle in an
exponential way, far above what you can do by yourself.

It is the last rep. It is the extra effort. It is finding
something in yourself that you didn't know you had. It is
wishing that you had put your stuff in a lower locker
because you can't reach the top one. It is being unable to
shampoo your hair because you can't reach that high, so
you bend over at the waist to give your arms a break.

You're there. You've been there for months. I can't
imagine what you've gone through. Part of me really
doesn't want to.

The Shawshank Redemption quote comes to mind:

"Andy crawled to freedom through five hundred yards of
shit smelling foulness I can't even imagine, or maybe I just
don't want to. Five hundred yards... that's the length of
five football fields, just shy of half a mile."

There's only one step left before you can be free of this
scourge. Eating like it is your job, even when you don't
feel like you can keep it down. Eat until failure. Then do it
again.

Keep doing what you are doing. I love you more than you
will ever know.

No retreat. No surrender. No compromise. You will beat this. You already have.

We need to pick a date for dinner.

July

7/1/12 - The path home

First, I want to tell you what a pleasure it was to spend time with you today, and to listen to the life in your voice, and to watch how animated you got when talking about what is going on at work.

You're on your way back. I don't know how I know this, but I do. Keep Believing in this fact with a capital B. It will not happen in a straight line, but it will happen.

I know you haven't been listening to the radio a lot lately, but one of the few songs that is being played on a regular basis (outside of Adele's entire catalog, which it is not possible to escape from), is a song by a band named "fun". The relevant stanza:

So if by the time the bar closes
And you feel like falling home
I'll carry you home tonight

Getting home has dominated my thoughts lately, especially in respect to your journey. I caught a showing of Apollo 13 earlier this week, and this quote stood out:

Jim Lovell: "Uh well, I'll tell ya, I remember this one time - I'm in a Banshee at night in combat conditions, so there's no running lights on the carrier. It was the Shangri-La, and we were in the Sea of Japan and my radar had jammed, and my homing signal was gone... because somebody in Japan was actually using the same frequency. And so it was - it was leading me away from where I was supposed to be. And I'm lookin' down at a big, black ocean, so I flip on my map light, and then suddenly: zap. Everything shorts out right there in my cockpit. All my instruments are gone. My lights are gone. And I can't even tell now what my altitude is. I know I'm running out of fuel, so I'm thinking about ditching in the ocean. And I, I look down there, and then in the darkness there's this uh, there's this green trail.

"It's like a long carpet that's just laid out right beneath me. And it was the algae, right? It was that phosphorescent stuff that gets churned up in the wake of a big ship. And it was - it was - it was leading me home. You know? If my cockpit lights hadn't shorted out, there's no way I'd ever been able to see that. So uh, you, uh, never know... what... what events are to transpire to get you home."

You're going to get home, Carla. I know this. Maybe it takes all of your cockpit lights going out to show you the path, but the path is there. Find it and follow it.

There is a way through. In the meantime, do not retreat. Do not surrender. Adapt, Improvise, and Overcome.

7/2/12 - Blog post

Kelly forwarded this to me. It is an excellent short article that I think you would get some benefit from. I know that it deepened my understanding with regards to what you are going through.

http://well.blogs.nytimes.com/2012/06/21/life-interrupted-fighting-cancer-and-myself/?src=rechp

7/2/12 - Living on a prayer

For whatever reason, the muses have not been talking to me tonight. They're probably taking the night off and watching the male stripper movie.

Whatever.

The important part is that you're halfway home. You've reached the watershed point. All of the rivers are now flowing in a different direction, and all of this is positive for you.

Be patient. Save your energy for the fights that matter. You can find a way through. In other words, keep doing what you've been doing. Eat like a 13 year old boy - I loved listening to you telling me about your late night kitchen raids. Keep that attitude up and you will get through.

I love you more than you can possibly know. Do not retreat. Do not surrender. No compromises.

I can't help myself - sorry for putting this into your head:

"Oh, we're halfway there...
Oh, living on a prayer..."

See you on Tuesday afternoon.

7/3/12 - Persistence

I quote myself, from February 2, my first day in Maui, and the end of your first week of chemo/radiation.

"Was reading the paper this morning and happened to see this in the horoscope section:

'Persistence in the face of failure is often the key to eventual success, except in skydiving.'

You're not skydiving."

We talked about the inevitability of physical symptoms today. Not a lot you can do about that. But you are still here. You've proven that you can do this. You can get through this.

You can't escape the handcuffs that you're locked in to, to take a line from the blog that I forwarded you. But resistance and persistence take many forms. Andy Dufresne tunneled through a prison wall in The Shawshank Redemption. There is no such thing as an impossible situation.

Draw upon your secondary source of spiritual fuel. Draw upon the people who visited today. Draw upon Stu and his parents. Draw upon the strength that The Naturopath provides, no matter how bad he is at IV's. Conserve your energy for the important things.

I know that it is difficult, but be patient. I knew in my bones that OLM would be a success when I first saw it. It took 3 years before the finances ever showed it. There is a picture of me in our old offices with a whiteboard in the background that says "Overnight 5 Year Success." I look fat. Many things change.

We're coming up on the 5-year anniversary of OLM selling out to ThyssenKrupp. Regardless of whether that was a good or bad idea, it is validation of our persistence, and the validity of our idea. You can do the same thing, although there will be a lot less lying to vendors about when exactly the check was mailed, and it will take a lot less than 3 years.

Trust in the process, Carla. I know that things seem bleak, but remain persistent. Believe in the outcome, and it can happen.

I love you more than you can possibly know.

Resistance comes in many forms. It does not necessarily need to be a frontal assault.

Adapt. Improvise. Overcome.

7/4/12 - Keep Believing

I've had a number of starts and stops today as I attempt to flesh out some ideas. In the meantime, this clip absolutely gives me chills every time I see it, not because of the immediate subject, (beating the dirty commies), but more for the overall message - miracles are possible, and they happen every day, even if they aren't recorded on video tape.

http://www.youtube.com/watch?v=8gfD134ED54&feature=youtube_gdata_player

I know for a fact that you don't need a miracle. You just need to stand your ground and let your body heal. Trust in the process. You just need to hold your territory. Read about the 101st Airborne and the defense of Bastogne if you're looking for kindred souls, or watch episodes 6-7 of Band of Brothers.

I know it feels like you are imprisoned by what you are going through, but your mind is freer than you can possibly imagine.

Keep adapting. Keep improvising. Keep overcoming. I'll see you in a couple of hours.

Text Messages: 7/5/12 12:44 PM

Carla: I am feeling so tired today. Sick too. Not sure I can make it. But please come at 300 today okay.

Me: I'll be there.

Carla: Thank u so much. Also could you get me sugar free jello pudding. Choc and vanilla. It's the only thing that sooths my throat.

7/5/12 - Focus

Ok. This is the most important one. This is the one you focus on. This is what you meditate on:

Yes. I'm motivating you with Rocky IV. No, I have no scruples. Just relax and work through it. You are going to survive. You are going to thrive.

Duke: All your strength, all your power, all your love. Everything you've got. Right now!

I could leave it at that. I probably should. But I believe in going over the top whenever possible.

Duke: You're gonna have to go through hell, worse than any nightmare you've ever dreamed. But when it's over, I know you'll be the one standing. You know what you have to do. Do it.

Duke: He's worried! You cut him! You hurt him! You see? You see? He's not a machine, he's a man!

Rocky: I see three of him out there.
Paulie: Hit the one in the middle.
Duke: Right! Hit the one in the middle.

Drago: [to his own trainer] He's not human. He's like a piece of iron.

Being scared is ok. That's what Stu and I are here for. Be a piece of iron. Do not give an inch. No compromises.

You can't hit the one in the middle, as much as you would like to.

What you can do is believe. You stopped the fistula with your Belief. Now it is time to stop cancer with that Belief.

You have already done it once. You can do it again.

I love you more than you can possibly imagine.

Adapt. Improvise. Overcome.

7/6/12 - The Law of Big Numbers

When I started at Copper & Brass Sales, way back in 1994, my trainer was a guy named Kevin. I bring this up only because you and I were talking about my propensity to see a situation and apply a movie quote to that situation. This behavior really had its origin with the year or so that I spent in the cubicle next to Reid.

If asked, he will claim that I'm better than him at the game. I will claim that he's better. In truth, we are both very, very good at it. This does not speak well of our social lives, but perhaps it has some purpose that we have not yet discerned.

But I'm not here to talk about movie quotes, or who can find the most relevant line from Caddyshack. I want to talk about what Kevin called the Law of Big Numbers.

You've probably heard a variation of this - "if an infinite number of monkeys sat in front of an infinite number of typewriters (or PC's running Word), how long would it take one of those monkeys to type out the full works of Shakespeare by pounding randomly on the keys?" My ex-wife was never strong on math and refused to accept the premise.

Reid and I had some really unbelievable debates as we were performing our drone/clerical work, until one day he threw out this thesis: "In an infinite Universe, anything that can happen, will, and probably already has."

Someday I'm going to smoke weed for the first time. I intend to meditate on that last statement for a very long time. And then eat a bag of Cheetos. And then a bag of Oreos Double Stuff. Because blood sugar spikes are a temporary thing. And a 12 year craving is impossible to describe.

More than that, I want you to think about something that The Naturopath told me once - we create by speaking. Our words can change reality. When you start thinking about the first chapter of Genesis, you'll have an aha moment. We create little worlds every time we speak.

Why am I talking about this? Because I want you to remember that in an infinite universe, anything is possible, and you can influence the course of events in the universe. The Law of Big Numbers states that everything, no matter how improbable, is possible.

I talked yesterday about the fact that you willed the fistula to go away. Now it is time to do the same with cancer. You can create your own reality. You can influence the universe with nothing more than your speech and your thoughts.

I love you more than you can possibly imagine.

Keep adapting. Keep improvising. Keep overcoming.

7/7/12 - In the beginning...

I talked a little bit yesterday about how The Naturopath once told me that we can create with our speech - what we say can become reality. I talked about the aha moment that I had with that from the first part of Genesis.

The aha moment really hits home when you think of the first sentence of the Gospel according to John: "In the beginning there was The Word." Think about that for a second. In the most spiritual of the Gospels, the first concept that is advanced is the primacy of speech.

I've been kind of obsessed with those twin concepts for a while, and I'm finally converting them to a physical reality.

Spent a good part of the afternoon Saturday getting worked on for the attached picture. The basic idea is that there is a banner coming out of the laptop on my arm. (Yes, I know, this is a weird sentence). On that banner will be 1's and 0's that spell out the sentence that I talked about. The banner will then morph into a strand of DNA.

Yes. Really Badass. And yet another way for me to continue to convince my nephew that I'm the coolest uncle ever, while horrifying Alice at the same time. It is the gift that keeps on giving, no matter how much the part on the inside my wrist hurt like a sonofabitch.

You have a similar power to make your words a reality. Create your future by speaking it. You've beaten the fistula by telling it that it was time to go. Do the same for whatever cancer cells remain in your body. Speak your future and make it happen.

Keep adapting. Keep improvising. Keep overcoming.

7/7/12 - Letter to Family / Friends

- Apparently, when an oncologist says that he recommends 4 rounds (6 weeks ago), what he really means is he wants 8 rounds (today). Math. Who knew it could be so complicated? She is not reacting well to yet another perceived failure to provide full information from her medical team.

She told me that even if her numbers were moving in the right direction the max she felt she could do was 6 rounds. As the victim/beneficiary of a personal trainer, I know she can do at least 7, and I think I can get her to 8, but I'm not going to do it unless there is some assurance that the juice is worth the squeeze.

- She's put on between 8-12 pounds, depending on the scale and her clothing, and won a $20 bet with Stu as a result. Degenerate gamblers are so much easier to motivate. A lot of this is due to the fact that she's eating like a 13 year old teenage boy, with all of the good and bad connotations that come from that statement.

- Mainly, she is really tired, as the chemo is kicking the crap out of her red blood cells.

At this point, we are collectively in a holding pattern - the next cancer marker test is scheduled for two Tuesdays from now. If things are holding steady or improving, she'll keep on doing chemo. If not, she's told me that she's done - it is just too difficult without some prospect of a positive outcome.

Thanks to all for listening.

PS - please welcome two new members to the email list, Rachele and Lisa, who for some reason have asked to be added to this tale of woe. My readership just went up by 25%!

Text Messages: 7/8/12 9:30 PM

Me: Looks like Wednesday works really well, unless it is better for Stu and his band practice on Thursday. I really like hanging out, whether we have deep conversations or not.

Me: New email sent, a little earlier than usual - I don't have a lot of control over the Muses - they speak to me on their own schedule, not mine.

Me: I love you more than you can possibly imagine. You're going to survive this.

7/8/12 - On the subject of not fighting

We talked a week or so ago about how what you're doing is not really fighting, but rather dealing with the arrivals of symptoms of going through chemo, and the subtle differences between the two reactions.

I found a couple of quotes that seemed to make sense to me in this area, and I wanted to pass them on to you. They are not perfectly on point, but they get close enough to the heart of the matter, and I know that you can make the intellectual leap to see how they apply.

The first one is tangentially related to a little bit of history between you and I, but if you expand past that, and see it in its entirety, I think it fits quite well:

Hawkeye in Last of the Mohicans: "No, you submit, do you hear? You be strong, you survive... You stay alive, no matter what occurs! I will find you. No matter how long it takes, no matter how far, I will find you."

I don't read this as me saying it. I look at in a larger spiritual context. Stay flexible. Accept what you can. Submit to what you cannot. But do not ever give up hope, no matter what your body is telling you. You can do this - save your energy and conserve your resources. Keep your eyes on the horizon. You will be found.

The other quote is from an obscure set of fantasy novels that I'm embarrassed to admit I've ever read. The story isn't bad, but overall they're basically popcorn for the brain. One quote, however, is important, from Kushiel's Dart:

"That which yields is not necessarily weak."

Where you have to accept the physical consequences of your treatment, do so. But don't confuse feeling like crap with failing. You are not weak, and yielding to physical symptoms that you have no control over is very different than giving in.

No compromises.

Keep adapting. Keep improvising. Keep overcoming.

Text Messages: 7/9/12 9:15 PM

Carla: It would be over the weekend. Sat/Sunday. Watch movies whatever. Just hang out.

Me: You can count on me being there. Love you!

Carla: Trying to stay awake and watch war games. Probably won't make it through.

Me: The code that Joshua finds at the end is CPE 1704 TKS.

Me: I am such a geek.

Carla: Yes you are!! Too funny.

7/9/12 - World Views

Your comment about watching WarGames triggered something that prompted me to connect some competing world views as expressed in popular culture. I know which one I pick. Which one do you choose?

From WarGames:

[after playing out all possible outcomes for Global Thermonuclear War]

Joshua: Greetings, Professor Falken.

Stephen Falken: Hello, Joshua.

Joshua: A strange game. The only winning move is not to play.

From The Wire:

Marla Daniels: You cannot lose if you do not play.

From Rounders:

Mikey: I told Worm you can't lose what you don't put in the middle. But you can't win much either.

Hard to believe, but it keeps coming back to one very simple concept that we've been talking about since almost the beginning of our relationship:

Do, or do not. There is no try.
If you want to be an actor, BE an actor.

You're either in or you're out. There are only so many ways to express this.

I'd like to point out that this dovetails with an argument we had a decade or so ago, about how ones and zeroes run the universe, and how yes/no decisions were really important.

You've shown, again and again, that you are capable of putting your chips in the middle. You never knew Fox, but I am certain that he would have approved. As his representative here, and as your friend, I am in awe. Your intestinal fortitude is on full display.

You've done some amazing, awesome work. There is more left to do.

There is a difference between acceptance and yielding. Find that space. Recognize that feeling like shit is not the same as giving in.

Do not compromise.

Keep adapting. Keep improvising. Keep overcoming.

More than anything - keep believing.

7/10/12 - Time Travel in Reverse

My love of time travel stories is well-documented. We only have to recount the fact that I saw The Lake House not once, but four times, to establish that.

I've imagined a lot of these scenarios over the years. I usually settle on going back to 1977, if only so I can watch Star Wars on the big screen at the drive in theater, and establish my bona fides with Fox by quoting from Jaws and The Godfather, decades before I saw them the first time around. I'm pretty sure that would have been enough to convince him that his 8 year old son was, in fact, a time traveler. Quoting the score of the Super Bowl was my ace in the hole. That and my extensive knowledge of swear words would probably be sufficient.

The basic plan that I've developed is to have a Come to Jesus conversation with him, but to cut Alice out of it entirely - as open as she is now to the weird stuff, in the late '70s and '80s, she was still firmly rooted in the 1950's. Fox was a gambler at heart, looking to eke some advantage from changing trends. He would understand.

In recent months, though, I've spent way less time thinking about becoming my 8 year old self, and how I would explain the situation to Fox, and more obsessed with conversations with my 53 and 63 year old self, 10 and 20 years in the future.

The point of this whole diatribe, I think, is to remind you that while the past is set, we are all still in control of our future. I know you feel like crap right now. This is not your future. You're going to survive. I know this on a level that I can't explain.

263

Assuming that fact, what would your future self say to you now? I think that "thank you for hanging in" would lead the list, but I want to hear your thoughts.

Keep adapting. Keep improvising. Keep overcoming.

I love you more than you can imagine.

7/12/12 - The squishy sound

I want to thank you from the deepest part of my heart for your two comments today, first, that me handling the pickups is important to you and helps you feel better, and second, that you know you can rely on me. You know who I am, and I hope you can appreciate how much both comments meant to me.

The business dinner ran long tonight - one of the guys just wouldn't shut up about all of the wonderful things he'd done in his career. Grrrrrrr. Into each life a little rain must fall.

Of course, that is but a minor annoyance, and the fact that it was happening at Daniel's Broiler tends to mitigate my anger, as I was in a meat stupor at the time.

Really looking forward to this weekend. I know you always apologize to me for falling asleep, or doing nothing more exciting than watching TV all day, but I want you to understand how much I enjoy these things. It isn't so much what we are doing than it is the fact that I can provide some level of comfort to you.

I've said it before, and I'll say it again - every time I visit, I feel like I am in the exact right place at the exact right time. It is enormously fulfilling for me.

You've known me for a long time. You know that I have a selfish tendency - part of the reason I got BJ was to prove to myself that I could care for something other than myself. Also, of course, because she's awesome. She's just this perfect Zen being who reminds me every day to live in the moment.

But I digress. I know that the price you are paying is high, but at least for me it has reawakened some level of my humanity that I shut down a long time ago. For whatever time I am involved in taking care or watching over you, I can extend myself in a way that I haven't been able to in a very long time, and it feels awesome.

I know that there are a lot of ways that would have been a lot easier on you to tap into this for me. But the fact remains that I've been the beneficiary of a great gift, and I want to thank you for your part in helping me to become more human.

Ok, way too much about me. Let's talk about you. Let's talk specifically about you in the summer of 1999, freaking out about speaking in front of 50 or 60 Fast Company geeks as part of the introduction of a guest speaker. Fast forward to five years later, when it wasn't even a blip on your radar to do the same thing in front of several hundred people. You thrived on doing that.

Here's the thing - people like us are really rare. We may fail in a given approach, but we keep getting up and running into the brick wall. Even when we hear the squishy sound after our skulls have given way. Because we know in our hearts that we are right in a way that is difficult to express to unbelievers. And we're going to keep adapting, improvising, and overcoming until we find a way through, over, around, or under that wall.

Or perhaps we will short-circuit the process by either refusing to admit that the wall exists, or figuring out a way to teleport around it.

During the times that we've run into the wall, it only appeared that we had failed. In truth, we had successfully found an idea that didn't work.

You know of my ridiculous love of Armageddon, which rivals your love of Road House. I maintain that this is

Michael Bay's opus, and I now own the Director's Cut to prove it.

One line stands out with respect to how I view you:

AJ: "Harry will do it. He doesn't know how to fail."

I've known you for a very long time, and if I know anything, I know that you don't know how to fail. I've seen it over the course of our relationship.

Rely on this aspect of your personality. You will find a way through. You will survive. You will not fail.

Keep improvising. Keep adapting. Keep overcoming.

I love you more than you can possibly imagine.

Text Messages: 7/12/12 12:05 PM

Me: Do not allow your anxiety to interfere with your faith.

Carla: Thank you for this it helps.

7/12/12 - The night that the muse did not speak

I really can't describe my process for sending you these emails. Basically, I get drunk and then send off what pops into my head, trusting that it will have some value to you.

This is my version of the wall that I talked about last night. Sometimes I go over the wall. Sometimes I go around. Sometimes I refuse to acknowledge that the wall exists.

I've trusted in this process for a very long time. The number of times that the Universe, or the Muses, have reached out to me is insanely large. There are no coincidences.

Tonight, though, I have nothing. Or maybe, by accepting that there are no coincidences, I have taken a step forward in understanding.

I don't have a silver bullet tonight. Hopefully you can understand that you are not alone, that there is something larger than what we see, and whatever it is wants to, in the end, see that you are happy.

Yes, I know. This all sounds like bullshit. But I think I'm on to something that I can't describe. I am looking forward to talking to you on Saturday.

Keep improvising. Keep adapting. Keep overcoming. I love you more than you can imagine

7/12/12 - From Carla, to me:

It's okay. Some of your emails last me for days. You don't have to have one every day. Send something when you feel inspired!! Looking forward to tomorrow.

Text Messages: 7/13/12 6:04 PM

Carla: Just keep in mind that I am super tired and might sleep most of the time you are here. Hope that's okay.

Me: Absolutely ok by me. I like being there to watch over you, even if you are fast asleep.

Carla: Thanks again for everything!!

Me: You're welcome. It was my pleasure. It is clear that you're on the road to a full recovery!

Carla: You think so. Someday I'm sure and other days like today I just don't know.

7/13/12 - Some Random Thoughts

Thanks for understanding about the inspiration thing.
The fact that a single email can last a couple of days is
humbling, but I'll keep it in mind as I try to deliver the
really good stuff, rather than something so-so.

There may be a second email tonight, but I'm not sure yet.
This one was sent out to the office this evening. We have a
Customer Service Team of 3 people who try to keep us all
focused on the goal.

To that end, they ran a contest where everyone submitted
their best customer service lines. I was completely
floored about how similar the lines were when the
answers were revealed.

That team then SuperGlued some trophies together out of
materials in our scrap bin. It was the most OLM thing
ever, and I was absolutely moved by the trophies, and the
approach that our people have. This is roughly equivalent
to the Secret Happiness Committee putting Matchbook
cars on every desk when you were at Perkins.

You'll recognize the style; I've been refining it for the last
decade or so, and have really nailed it in the last seven
months. You even have a cameo role. With that, enjoy
what your pupil has become, because I couldn't have
written any of this without your help.

You're going to get back to doing this kind of work, Carla.
I know it, in a way I cannot express, and I want you on our
team when it happens. With that as prelude...

Team -

I've been thinking for the last several hours about the Best Customer Service Line Ever contest and awards that were handed out on Friday.

First, thanks to the Customer Service Team for leading this initiative, and for coming up with such unique awards. In the last couple of weeks, I've received a couple of awards for being with ThyssenKrupp for 5 years - one was a lucite-encased piece of paper, the other a $30 pair of binoculars. None of these means as much to me, or exemplifies what OLM is about, than the ones that were handed out today, both on an emotional and physical level.

When I first saw what was going on at Amber's desk, I will admit to feeling kind of disappointed. My cynical side (what? I have a cynical side?) said that this was a participation award, like every third grader receiving a ribbon just because they took part in some mini-race.

But the more I thought about it, and after hearing everyone's answers, the more I realized how appropriate this was. Each of us take our own individual approaches, but we're all working toward the same goal, which John and I recognized early on would be the lifeblood of our business: if you treat customers the way that you would want to be treated, they'll keep giving you money.

Carla and I have a shorthand term that we've used for this over years: "Money and Peace." It comes from a line in the movie Field of Dreams: "Sure, you can look around, you'll say. It's only $20. And they'll hand over the money because it money they have and it is peace that they lack." Those 3 sentences have been the core of what we've tried to build here at OLM. Solve a customer's problem and they will keep coming back.

Of course, we're not helping our customers achieve a higher plane of existence. We're selling metal (and plastics, and if John has his way, drill bits and mops and, I don't know, ball bearings (it's all ball bearings these days, as Fletch quite correctly pointed out)). We've said, over the years, that we're not actually selling metal and plastics and ball bearings - we're selling customer service and tossing the metals and plastics and ball bearings in for free.

Here's the thing - every single one of the answers to this contest reflected that simple fact. Maybe we've collectively built a company where that is the norm, and it isn't just paid lip service. Maybe it is just part of each of your natures. I really don't care. I'm just incredibly proud to be associated with it.

The coming years will have a lot of growth and a lot of change. We are approaching the elbow in the exponential curve. Each of you are going to play a key role in that growth - much as Money and Peace was the core of our approach to customers, you will collectively form the core of the team that takes care of those customers. Even the ones who are scared of using the Internet.

Thanks to the Customer Service team for creating these awards, which, with their SuperGlue and Duct Tape approach to design, and their simple, elegant messages, are the most tangible representations of the OLM Way that I've ever seen. I really hope that we can continue using these in the future - they are just uniquely OLM.

Thanks, most of all, to each of you, for doing the hard stuff every day, and for helping to build an environment where the exchange of Money for Peace is a lot less cynical than it might initially sound, and where the desire to give the customer a little Peace is what drives us.

Text Messages: 7/14/12 7:59 PM

Carla: Please be sure to tell your aunt thank you for me. It was so kind of her to think of me.

Me: I already have. Remember that you have a lot of people pulling for you. That kind of positive energy will absolutely help you - tap into it and feel its power.

Carla: I know and it is a source of great comfort. It always overwhelms me when it comes from people I don't even know.

7/14/12 - Coincidences and Pattern Recognition

OK. After today, I think I have a better understanding of how you're doing. I'm going to take a brief detour tonight as I process today's events. As my best friend, you're the person I want to discuss this stuff with.

This is from an email conversation from my Uncle Chad (my Aunt Kazuko's husband), who has been acting as my spiritual Godfather since about 1987. Most of this will be familiar to you, but this is the first time I've put it all down in one place.

First - his statement / question:

"I just tried to scan for you a chapter from psychiatrist Scott Peck's 'A Different Drum'. He talks about the stages of spiritual growth. Scanning took too long so I will send it via regular mail. He may help in the understanding of your situation. I don't want to summarize because I would over simplify it and destroy it.

"It seems like you used to be at the stage that 'if you can't scientifically prove what it is, then it doesn't exist, and stop talking nonsense and leave me alone' (kinda Ludwig Wittgenstein and Logical Positivism) but are at the stage that you think there is 'something out there' besides what you can feel/touch/see/prove but you don't know what it is or how it impacts your life.

"So what patterns and coincidences are you seeing? "

My response, off the top of my head:

Sports-related -

- Tebow's 316 yard game against the Steelers in the playoffs.

- Tebow's 31.6 yards per pass average in the same game.

- http://deadspin.com/5893117/the-shocking-proof-that-tim-tebow-and-tebowing-are-cosmically-linked. Basically, Tebow was born on the same day that a movie that included a Tebowing scene was released.

- Linsanity, from the perspective that he's also very Christian.

- The Immaculate Reception. Because why not?

These fall more into the pattern-recognition area; they serve to enhance a general awareness that something is going on.

Personal anecdotes -

- My absolute certainty that my grandmother was nearby during the three root canals that I underwent in the summer following her passing and was helping to calm me down. That could be chalked up to the nitrous oxide, of course.

- The story of my meeting a girlfriend-to-be (The Formerly Fair Kathryn) under the most improbable set of circumstances possible. That story would take a whole other email to explain.

- The entire ex-girlfriend and girl next door saga. This entire experience a) led me to meeting The Naturopath, b) set me on a road of self-discovery, c) prepped me for the Carla experience, and d) made me recognize, finally, the value of putting myself out there (as opposed to waiting for the perfect situation).

- The sudden insight that I wouldn't have been in a position to connect The Naturopath and Carla had I not done the stuff in the last bullet point. She would have had to go through this with only Western Medicine, and I'm convinced she very likely would not have made it this far except for his timely intercessions on her behalf.

- The fact that had I not transferred to Seattle, I was about to be transferred to Pittsburgh to take over the outside sales territory that Fox had patrolled when he was at Pennsylvania Industrial, a company that was purchased by Copper & Brass Sales in 1984.

- A conversation with Carla back in 2002 or so, where I asserted that everything could be represented with ones and zeroes, if you had a long enough string of ones and zeroes. The Universe generally follows a logical structure. Carla's assertion that ones and zeroes could not represent love. My eventual recognition that ones and zeroes cannot represent two things - Null (the absence of any value) and Infinity. Pair that with the Alpha and Omega statement and you've got a weird alignment of concepts across 2,000 or so years.

The idea that we are in Purgatory is not by any means a new one. Similarly, the Buddhists, from what (very) limited understanding I have, view the concept of multiple lives as a way that the Universe helps us to keep getting closer to Nirvana, little by little.

From those two perspectives, the appearance of Jesus in history could be interpreted as (forgive the imperfect computer metaphor) God or the Universe or whatever providing a programming shortcut to get past the concept of having to wait for a huge number of lives to have passed before approaching Nirvana. Still working to flesh out this idea.

If you'll remember, I have on my right forearm a tattoo of a hand coming out of a computer and pressing the keys. I spent last Saturday expanding it, (something that I'm sure will freak Alice out as a secondary benefit).

Out of the computer, there comes a banner that scrolls up and down my forearm. On that banner are ones and zeroes, which, if we read binary easily, would translate to "In the Beginning there was the Word." Eventually, the banner splits, and resolves itself into a strand of DNA (the building blocks of life itself) that wraps itself around my wrist. It really does look awesome.

Anyway, that's just the prologue. It was during my two hours on the table that I had a personal insight that ties back into a) the Purgatory thing, above, and b) your statement about parents making us eat our vegetables.

She was in the process of working on the inside of my wrist. I really can't describe how much this hurt - the skin is very thin, and it is basically right on top of the bone, and the fact that it was long straight lines just added to the discomfort level. It hurt so much that I was seriously considering stopping and going through the rest of my life with a half-finished tattoo.

Charlie gave me a piece of advice - "This is actually easier for you if you relax, no matter how hard that is to do." That triggered memories of conversations that I've had with The Naturopath about acceptance and attachment (he leans Buddhist, with some Lakota Indian thrown in - really interesting guy. I have an alternate theory about him that doesn't fit into this narrative), and conversations with Carla about the fact that you don't really fight cancer or chemo - you accept that the side effects are going to show up no matter what you do.

I came to see the tattoo experience as a pretty good metaphor for life and spirituality, if you accept either the Purgatory Premise or the Buddhism Premise at their most basic. In order to get to a more perfect You (or, in this case, to have some badass body art), you're going to have to go through some pain that is more than you think you can bear.

Continuing the metaphor, there are any number of tools that we can use to handle this pain, and I went through all of them. Meditating and trying to discern each individual needle strike rather than the pain that it caused (Buddhist); focusing on the end result of an awesome tattoo (Christian-ish); submission to the will of Charlie (mostly Islam, but without the kneeling 5 times a day and the blowing up of infidels or the rejection of bacon as the most perfect food ever). I couldn't come up with something suitable for Judaism, mainly because I started thinking too much about how much I like bacon. Ditto for the Hindus, because you can take my ribeye steak away from me when you pry it from my cold, dead hands.

I'm not yet ready to commit to one particular path - I've come to see that there are multiple ones. I think that the important thing for me is that the idea that we're born and we live a comparatively short life, and then there is nothing but oblivion afterwards has been effectively put to rest.

I could've solved this problem a lot earlier if I had just listened to Yoda in The Empire Strikes Back:

"Luminous beings are we, not this crude matter."

There is a phenomenon (not sure the name of it) that basically says that if, for instance, you buy a Volvo, all the sudden you'll start noticing every Volvo on the road as you're driving. I willingly stipulate that this explains some of what I'm experiencing and seeing - if you look hard enough, you can make a coincidence out of anything. The vast number of coincidences leads me to the conclusion that there is something else that can't be accounted for by random number theory.

The patterns are out there, and the coincidences keep piling up. If not for the fact that I was terrible in stats class (ironic, given what I do for a living), I'm sure that I could come up with some probabilities, and they would quickly approach the asymptotic line.

Text Messages: 7/15/12 11:37 AM

Me: I have a suggestion. Instead of focusing on your anxiety this week, focus instead on your faith. Focus on the belief that has gotten you this far.

Me: It isn't your body that is being tested. It never has been. It is your faith. I can't say why, but your faith and your belief will sustain you.

Me: I love you more than you can possibly imagine. Keep adapting. Keep improvising. Keep overcoming. But most of all, keep believing.

Me: All I ask is that when you get anxious, to rely on your Faith and your Belief.

Me: You can do this. Look at what you have already done. Look at what you've overcome. You've done a lot more with a lot less.

Carla: I'm trying. As Tuesday gets closer it just gets a bit harder.

Me: I know. This is the time to practice your breathing.

7/15/12 - A blast from the past

Let's talk about a conversation from a lifetime ago, when you had just met Stu and were full of anxiety. Do you remember my response?

Before you answer, here's the rest of the story - while listening to you on that day, way back in 2002, I remembered a movie quote from Bull Durham:

"Don't think, Meat. It can only hurt the ball club." You were thinking way too much and not just letting things happen. That's why I came up with an approach that worked for you:

Be the boy.

That was less about your status in the relationship than it was about taking control of your feelings and emotions.

You've done this before. You can do this again. Take control of your feelings and emotions. Be the boy where necessary.

Above all, rely on your Faith and your Belief. It will sustain you.

7/16/12 - A little bit of inspiration

In yet another case of the cosmic tumblers clicking into place and the Universe opening up and showing us what is possible, my friend Bridget Lyons posted this today. You'll remember her as the one who recommended a raw food diet almost immediately after you were diagnosed.

A fair amount of what she says is specific to her life, but there is a large section that applies directly to you, and the things that we've been talking about.

I have a gut feeling and profound hope that this will provide you with what you need right at this moment. The product of Faith and Belief is Grace, or so I was taught growing up.

http://theyogadiaries.net/2012/07/16/open-to-grace-are-you-serious/

I love you more than you can possibly imagine. Keep trusting in your Faith and your Belief. Let the Universe help you through the gift of Grace.

Text Messages: 7/16/12 10:02 PM

Carla: Thank you for your email tonight. It really helps to keep me focused and positive.

Me: I got lucky. Bridget posted that on Facebook an hour ago. The Universe continues to smile on you, Carla.

Me: In my left brained way, this makes sense: Faith x Belief = Grace. Grace can solve a lot of things.

Me: You can do this. I love you.

Carla: I agree and this could not have come at a better time.

Carla: You are channelling a lot of powerful things from the universe to me. Thank you.

Me: I'm just a conduit. All I'm trying to do is stay open to anything that will help you.

Me: And I'm not above cheating and/or stealing the ideas of others. You're worth it.

Me: Keep your head up. The Universe is working for you. Focus on Grace tonight. I have a feeling that that concept is important.

Carla: I couldn't agree more.

7/17/12 - Surviving the perp walk

One of the enduring images on TV news is the Perp Walk. It is a subtle way of shaming those accused and/or convicted of crimes. The subjects are led, their hands cuffed behind their backs, utterly helpless, to a waiting car. Most try to hide their faces.

There is, of course, no good security reason for doing this. Jack Ruby made that point 50 years ago. We do it as a lesson to others - Society has decided that shaming those who likely committed crimes is an effective way of encouraging others not to commit crimes.

You know that the likelihood of me showing up in a Perp Walk is so remote as to be infinitesimal, but it remains one of my great fears - being innocent of a crime, and forced to make the Ultimate Walk of Shame, knowing the friends, family, acquaintances, and people I never even met would be judging me based on 15 seconds of video.

Have you ever noticed that the cameras always seem to catch at least a glimpse of the cuffs, to emphasize the fact that the criminal has been removed from polite society? At some level, it serves to tell both Society and the criminal that they are lesser people, that they are animals and deserve to be put in a cage.

Yes, I know. Pretty dark, but it ties in to something Earl was talking about today - our societal reaction to illness, especially cancer, is not usually favorable to the victims. Before all of this happened to you, if I saw a woman wearing a bandanna, or an obviously gaunt man with a bald head, my initial reaction was to pull back and to avert my eyes. I'm not proud of that.

Our treatment of the sick amongst us is shameful. We should be celebrating their courage and their resolve.

As I was driving to come pick you up today, I was stopped at an intersection where a woman wearing a bandanna was having difficulty getting across the street. Now that I've seen what it takes to get someone to that point, I would've waited all afternoon for her to get through the crosswalk.

I tell you this in order to establish a single fact: you getting out of the car, wearing the bandanna, and willingly walking in to Talarico's was easily the bravest act I've ever seen. I know you've been through a lot, and you've done things that are way harder, but I have a sense of how difficult it was for you to summon the courage to do that particular Perp Walk, and I feel honored to have seen it.

There is no reason for you to be confined to your room. You deserve to spread your wings and to venture out into the world. You're going to do it under your own power, and in small bites at first, but you need to see a world beyond your bedroom. I can be there whenever you want an assistant (or a partner in crime), and I don't particularly care if it lasts 5 minutes of 5 hours.

Turning to another subject - I know you are anxious about the marker number tomorrow. I'm anxious about the same thing, and I want you or Stu to tell me as soon as you know.

But remember what The Naturopath told you early on about that number - basically, chemo screws it up, as it is a measure of inflammation. It doesn't say definitively that something's going wrong. A couple of points in either direction are something to pay attention to, but they are not cause for panic (or, sadly, for celebration).

In short, don't panic. Don't obsess. It is an important test, but it is by no means definitive.

Think about what your body has done over the past 6 weeks and how it has responded. Think about the fact that it is growing hair in your nether regions after being burned by radiation. You are recovering. You are healing. Who gains weight on chemo? You do. Whose body expends energy on growing hair in an area nobody usually sees? Yours does, because the other stuff is under control.

Chemo has lived up to its marketing brochure so far. But you are still here. You're really tired, both emotionally and physically, but you're still here, and you keep looking better every time I see you.

I know and understand why you are focusing on the number tomorrow. I admit to doing the same thing. Don't let it define you. Don't let it dominate your emotions.

Next subject - spirituality. I don't even know where to begin, mainly because I am still trying to understand the about-face that I'm going through. As much as I would like to have this conversation via email, so that I can remove the emotion and deal with it dispassionately, it is really something that should be done in person.

Last, but not least - if you're looking for something to do on Saturday, I will be doing the rest of the tattoo from 12-3 on Saturday. Come and watch me cry like a little girl from 2:30 on, and we can go across the street to have a post-tattoo cocktail/mocktail.

I love you more than you can imagine. Keep finding a way, even if it means doing nothing at all.

Text Messages: 7/18/12 6:34 AM

Carla: Fuck. What a difference a day makes. I don't feel so good. Fuck fuck fuck. Saying fuck makes me feel better somehow.

Me: Sorry to hear that. But you made progress yesterday. Remember that you're healing, and that doesn't happen in a straight line.

Me: Use the tools you've learned to try to feel better. And by all means say the word Fuck as often as necessary.

Text Messages: 7/18/12 5:44 PM

Carla: Cea 9.0 down from 10.5 Just got the results.

Me: That is outstanding news. Congratulations!!!

Me: Keep trusting in your Faith. This won't be easy, but you are winning.

Carla: Well I know that is good news but that means that I have to keep doing this. I will for as long as it works it just means I feel like crap for another two months.

Me: Beats the hell out of the alternative.

7/18/12 - Inflection points

Ok. Today was kind of a big deal. I know, in talking to you, and watching your body language, how worried you were that the number had gone up.

But it didn't. It went down. The things that your body has been telling you - the extra energy, the appetite, the alertness, were correct. That's the good news.

The flip side, of course, is the fact that there is still a slog ahead of you. You've gotten notice of your parole, but it is two months away, and you are still in prison. You still have to get through 60 days.

This reminds me of a scene from The Princess Bride:

Fezzik: You just shook your head... doesn't that make you happy?

Westley: My brains, his steel, and your strength against sixty men, and you think a little head-jiggle is supposed to make me happy?

You know that I don't lie to you. The coming weeks will be difficult, but no more difficult than what you have already done. It will be a grind, but I know you. I know you can see it through. It is not too far.

I'm going to be right beside you the entire time, as will the rest of your staggeringly large entourage.

I know that this is a small thing, but I want to thank you for making me a part of your first non-medical foray in a lot of months on Tuesday. I have a sense of what it took for you to get out of the car. I wish it could have been more of a storybook ending, but real life doesn't always work that way. But you still did it. You took those steps.

You have my everlasting respect for having the fortitude to even try. That's what tells me that you're going to win. Your battle isn't physical. It isn't mind over matter. It is about acceptance and faith and grace. It is about finding a way to manage side effects and to find a way through.

I know that this message has veered away from the spiritual track that we were on; we'll get back to that soon, if only because I've recently realized how important it is. For now, trust what you've learned and trust that your path will open up as you walk it.

I love you more than you can possibly imagine. Keep improvising. Keep adapting. Keep overcoming.

Continue to rely on Faith. It can sustain you.

7/18/12 - Letter to Family / Friends

Let's cut straight to the heart of the matter - very good news just happened.

- The cancer marker test came in about an hour ago. The previous one was 10.5, the one from today is 9.0, so very good news. I'm not sure how good as I don't understand the scale, but Carla will see The Naturopath tomorrow and we'll get more knowledge of the implications.

- Given that she had convinced herself that it would be in the 20's, this is outstanding news, if only as a shot for her morale. I'll have a better read on that when I take her to see The Naturopath.

- Physically, she's looking a lot better, and is weighing in at nearly 130, up from a low of 112. I went over on Saturday and we grilled hamburgers - I made 2 for me and one for her; I wasn't fast enough and she grabbed the second one, then polished it all off with a pretty good sized piece of cake.

- Now that she's figured out how to manage the nausea (lots of ginger, lots of pot, one mild anti-nausea drug), she's an eating machine. She had a couple of slices of leftover pizza later in the afternoon.

- She is starting to see some hair loss, and has taken to wearing a bandana (thanks Kaz - it actually looks really good!) and she's pretty self-conscious about how she looks, which made what happened on Tuesday even more remarkable.

- I picked her up from chemo on Tuesday afternoon. Normally she just falls asleep in the car and goes straight to bed. This time, for the first time, she told me she didn't want to go into the house, so we spent 45 minutes driving all over West Seattle, where she pointed out a little park that she and her friends used to go to when she was in high school and could steal some beer from their parents.

- The capper came when we were driving down the main street in West Seattle and she had me park. We got out, walked up and down the block, then got back into the car and went home. This was her first time out of the house and not on her way into a hospital in about seven months, and even as self-conscious as she was about her hair and the tubes coming out of her, this was an enormous step forward.

- The implication of the positive test results is that she's going to feel like crap for the next two months as she does all 8 rounds, but that beats the hell out of the alternative, and I'm quite convinced, after seven months of emails, that I and others can keep her motivated enough to make it possible for her to get through it.

Thanks as always for reading.

Text Messages: 7/19/12 6:52 AM

Carla: It really means that I will need serious help for the next 8 weeks. Stu's parents leaving will be rough. You in?

Me: Fuck and yes.

Carla: It might mean more than picking me up from the dr office. Can u spare a bit more time in the coming weeks?

Me: I know. I want you to know that you can rely on me. I will make it work.

Carla: Thank you. I know that I would not have come this far without Stu's parents help so I need to be sure that I can fill some of the gaps that they provided.

Me: Whatever it takes, Carla. Whatever it takes.

7/19/12 - The power of speech

First, thanks for being so open with me today about the things that are dominating your thoughts and emotions. I can't imagine you doing anything else, but it was gratifying that you trusted me with your fears. Please continue to do so - as you said, I am, for whatever reason, channeling some good stuff lately, but it really helps if you tell me where you are so that I can help direct the channel a little bit.

I'm going to zig a little bit here - I have the beginnings of a master plan to help you, based largely on some things that The Naturopath taught me. It will take me a couple of days to work it out in my mind, and all I ask is that you trust me when we move forward with it.

I am going to admit that I was not completely forthcoming with you about the reason I'm seeing The Naturopath next week, and what we talk about. It will largely be preventative maintenance, but the fact that the ex is coming into town at the beginning of August and is having a baby shower / party right next door on a Sunday is, I'm sure, an area that we will explore.

The point is that no matter how you work (and I have worked, believe me), to eliminate attachment to something, or to someone, or to an outcome, only sociopaths or people who live in Tibet can cut the attachment cleanly. It will remain with you. The ex-girlfriend attachment is not going to magically disappear if I meet someone, fall in love, and settle down. It will approach an asymptotic curve, but it will never be eliminated entirely. But it no longer dominates my destiny. It can be the same for you as well.

In Yoda-speak: "Once you start down the Dark path, forever will it dominate your destiny."

292

In Fox-speak: "You can't unscramble those fucking eggs." "You can't put the shit back in the donkey." "White-out shows weakness."

Luke-speak: "No. I am a Jedi, like my father before me."

Sypolt-speak: "I really, really need to build a time machine."

Staring down attachment is a scary, difficult thing, even when the thing you are staring down is a scary thing that you don't want to remember. But it is a case where the mind is more powerful than the matter, and you have plenty of reserves in this area.

This is a chance to take all the powerlessness that you've felt over the past 7 months, all the helplessness you feel when you walk into the hospital again, all the fear that you've had at 3 am, and channel it into removing the power that an incorrect diagnosis - and that's what I truly believe it was - has over you.

Read that last paragraph again. I'll wait.

Ok. Read it again. Seriously.

Keep reading it. You have a chance to get even. You have a chance to direct your energy and your power in a way that will actually benefit you, rather than struggling against something over which you have no control.

The diagnosis was a thought. A thought has no power unless we take steps to empower it. It is vaporous and without substance.

Look at how many things they've been wrong about. Weaning you off the meds in the hospital by cutting you off cold turkey, because that's the protocol, comes to mind. I'm sure that you can think of a lot of others.

Their diagnosis was flat out wrong. You may discount The Naturopath's conversation about the pulses, but I absolutely believe every single word of it. If he isn't feeling anything, there is nothing there to feel.

You could probably stop chemo now, but you've developed a routine for managing the side effects that seems to work for you. The next 4 rounds are about insurance, about removing the smallest chance that Herman Jr. is still lurking. Don't give him a fucking chance. Club those baby seals. Every single last one of them.

I've talked about a basic technique for breathing before that The Naturopath gave me - inhale while speaking the word "Bliss", exhale while speaking the word "Attachment". Let's start with that, but substitute "Health" or "Healing" for "Bliss".

I have a couple of extra steps that I want you to go through, but let's start there. When you feel your anxiety rising about the subject of the misdiagnosis, take the time to breathe and to speak, and remember that you create with your speech. Keep your focus on creating, and always remember one thing:

In The Beginning There Was The Word.

Keep adapting. Keep improvising. Keep overcoming. I love you more than you can possibly imagine.

Text Messages: 7/20/12 11:03 PM

Me: No great insights tonight, at least that I can convert to written form. Looking forward to spending Saturday evening with you.

Carla: Okay. Then your punishment is to make me hamburgers for dinner!! Agreed!

Me: Deal!

Carla: Okay but I will also need the baked chips to truly make the meal complete

Me: Duh!

7/23/12 - A good walk spoiled (I'll explain later)

First, I want you to know and understand something that I was trying to communicate when I sent you my schedule last night.

You are my first priority. There are some things that I can't get out of, but you know how seriously I take commitments, especially when you're involved.

You're my favorite person in the whole world, so at some level this is a selfish thing (I like spending time with you and want to see you healed), but I want to reiterate something I've said in the past - when I come over, it feels so natural, so right, so effortless to be there. I can't explain it easily.

Actually, there was one other time in my life that I've felt this. It involves golf, but bear with me. Don't discount the feeling because of where it happened.

In the summer of 1998, my marriage was falling apart, and I knew it. Since I had nothing else to do after work, I spent a lot of time on a local course that charged $4 for all you could play after 4 pm. Even when walking, I could easily get in 27 holes.

I played a lot with a guy named Scott back then. He worked in the CBS purchasing department; I had at that point transferred to the sales group. We went out one Friday, and nothing went right. I lost balls in the middle of the fairway. If the hole bordered on out of bounds, I could be assured that my drive would find it. The more I tried to guide my shots, the worse they got.

I ended up shooting a 76 for 9 holes. To put this in perspective, at that point my typical score on this course was 42-46 for 9 holes. Pure frustration.

I went out the next day (a Saturday) at 4 pm, since I had nothing better to do, Netflix hadn't been invented, and I had a slow dial up connection that made porn agonizingly slow to download. Don't judge me. Ok, judge me.

I bogeyed the first hole (one over par), which was unusual for me. I usually owned the first hole - it was a short par five that I was usually able to reach in two. Not this time. Great, I thought. A continuation of yesterday.

And then something amazing happened. I ended up playing 36 holes that day. I looked at my scorecard after the 35th hole, and realized that with the exception of the first hole, I had just played 34 holes at par.

Of course, once I realized that fact, I tensed up and took a bogey on the final hole, mainly because I yanked an easy two foot putt.

I have never approached the feeling of being in the right place at the right time since - those 34 holes were transcendent. There was no effort at all; it was as easy as breathing.

Since then, I've been looking for that feeling, and the only place I've found it over the past 7 months is in 2 places. The main time I feel it is when I'm at the house. Every so often, I hit it when writing these emails.

My muse seems to have picked up stakes recently - no matter how much I call upon her, the raw inspiration that I've been channeling isn't there for the past couple of nights. In its place is something a bit more subtle which I am having trouble quantifying and/or translating.

The story that I just told is 100% true, and when I've thought about it in the days since, it tells me that the

Universe has some holes in it. I believe that they were deliberately placed in order to show us what is possible when we relax and let our natural selves take over.

I'm pretty sure that you've found one or two of these holes along the way. They exist to help us believe. They exist to remind us that there is something larger that we can't perceive, but which is actively working to make us happy.

Be aware of these things. Yes, I do know that I'm the last person that you would have expected to espouse these beliefs.

You asked me, about 8 weeks ago, if I believed in God. I told you yes, because that's what I knew you needed to hear, even when I didn't believe. I'm not proud of that.

But I've seen too much in the past 8 weeks to deny the existence of a Universe larger than myself. I'm not ready to put a label on what it is; the Catholic in me wants to call it God, but whatever it is, it is far more subtle than an old guy with a beard.

What does this have to do with you? You live in a world where God is still performing miracles. They are really subtle - I still can't explain my golfing experience in 1998. God switched tactics from things like burning bushes, but He is still there, and He is watching over us. Unless, of course, Kevin Smith was right, and God looks like Alanis Morisette, in which case it is ok to reverse the pronouns.

Trust in that.

And yes, I can't believe that I've written the last couple of paragraphs. As I've said before, it has been a year of firsts. I hope that you know me well enough to realize that I am only saying these things because I really believe them.

Keep adapting. Keep improvising. Keep overcoming.

I love you more than you can possibly imagine.

7/24/12 - There, it's out!

I look back at my emails from time to time, if only to remember what I wrote. I'm recognizing a trend lately, and that's that I'm writing more about myself than about you. At some level, this is probably deliberate - as you said when we were at GroupHealth, it is remarkable to see the changes that I've made (or that have happened to me, depending on your perspective), and as you once told me, these emails are as therapeutic for me as they are, at some level, inspirational for you.

I freely admit that I don't really know where a lot of it is coming from. I have a couple of drinks and think about what I've seen that day or in previous weeks, and I try to connect the dots. It seems to work more often than it doesn't.

Went to see The Naturopath today. Originally, this was just supposed to be preventative maintenance, but a lot of the conversation revolved around my insight during the tattoo session a couple of weeks ago. He jokingly suggested that he should sum up the visit on my chart with "Found God". I told him that he wasn't that far off. Cannot possibly describe how differently I view the world since that moment of insight, as well as the subsequent ripples that have occurred.

Back to strictly physical matters, I've had a problem in my right buttock that kept getting worse over the last couple of months - a deep knot in the muscle that was affecting every muscle in my upper leg and some as far away as mid-calf.

The Naturopath found the knot (not difficult, as it was about the size of a softball) and also pointed out that my right hamstring was as tight as anything he'd ever seen, which explained the pain I had been experiencing. The big

300

relief for me is that it isn't structural. Fox had both hips replaced, and Alice has sciatica, both of which are hereditary. Looks like both of those are off the table for now.

He did the needle thing, then pulled out his Big Book of Chinese Wisdom. Based on the points he identified, this correlates to spending too much energy holding back from jumping on an opportunity. Not sure what that means, as there aren't a lot of opportunities that have come my way.

I don't mean that the way that it sounds - I'm really blessed in a lot of ways, and I recognize that. It is more that other than my sudden realization that there is a God, not a lot has been going on that could be called an opportunity. Then again, maybe I need to reexamine that last sentence.

In an unusual turn of events, we didn't spend a lot of time talking about you. Our conversations have always been pretty one-way, where I report how I view how you're doing, and he nods a lot. I understand completely - you deserve your privacy.

I talked about your attachment to the diagnosis from a couple of months ago, and how I perceive that it has impacted you. His response: "Fuck that doctor. You put 10 docs in a room and you're going to get 11 diagnoses. Maybe 15, if too many lawyers are involved."

A couple of thoughts -

First, I understand completely why that diagnosis continues to dominate your emotions and your imagination. If I were you, I'd be doing much the same thing.

You are my best friend. I feel deeply for you as you have to deal with hearing that diagnosis. My diagnosis kept me up for a couple of nights so I have a very minimal understanding of what you are feeling. I imagine that what the doc said to you keeps you up most nights. This is life-changing shit that you're dealing with. It need not dominate your destiny, however.

Don't want to get newly mystical with you, but there is a Zen koan that deals directly with this problem (my knowledge of this one goes back to an Eastern Religions class in 1990, so this is not something I've recently come to):

Q: If there is a goose trapped in a bottle, how do you get the goose out without breaking the bottle or killing the goose?

A: There, it's out!

The lesson, I think, is that situations that we believe to be untenable can be reversed without regards to the mechanics of how the reversal occurs. This really applies to our emotional health - sometimes all it takes is a good night's sleep, sometimes it takes a little longer, but outlooks can change quite suddenly. I've experienced it, and I know for a fact that you will too.

The second thought is a corollary to the Tattoo Insight. This one goes way off the reservation, but I can't come up with an argument to refute it. The fact that I can't come up with evidence to support it, other than pure conjecture, argues against it. Still, it is intriguing.

The Tattoo Insight, stated simplistically, says that we are here to absorb some pain in order for our souls to grow or to become more beautiful (the end result of the tattoo pain is an awesome tattoo; the end result of a life that has challenges is a soul that is more perfect and closer to God).

John was bitching today because he had to get a whooping cough shot due to his kids. Amber chirped in with the fact that she'd spent 90 minutes in the dentist's chair. I not so politely pointed out that I'd spent upwards of 5 hours in hands of Charlie the Terrible, without anesthetic.

John's response: yeah, but that was elective.

My response: that didn't stop it from fucking hurting a lot.

So the question I have, formulated at 3 pm on a Tuesday, when I was stone sober, is this: What if, before we were born, we chose our paths? What if we decide that our souls are getting a tattoo, no matter what it takes?

My moment of decision during the tattoo was this - I had to determine which was worse: gutting my way through the tat, with whatever tools I had available, or leaving with a half-finished tat, looking like an idiot?

What if our souls have made the same calculations, and asked the same questions? What if our souls have charted a course for us that is both fraught with danger, and enormously rewarding if we can pull it off?

I freely admit that this is nebulous and the result of pure speculation. It is not The Answer. It is An Answer, and there is a good chance that it is the wrong one. That only means it is worth further exploration.

My gut tells me that I am on to something. I'd really like to hear your thoughts.

7/25/12 - Email From Carla

This is one of the best ones you've sent so far. Thank you. These emails are priceless and mean more to me than you know.

7/25/12 - Transitions

I'll admit that after yesterday, I'm feeling spiritually spent. The implications of the Corollary to the Tattoo Insight have my brain reeling a little bit. It fits with my experience in so many ways, but there is precisely zero to support it. At least so far. But I know that I'm on to something.

I want to try to help you detach yourself a little bit from the diagnosis and all of the emotions and fears that you associate with it. The Naturopath's suggestion about writing about everything you feel about the diagnosis, as well as your fears, and then burning those pages, is absolutely sound. He had me do that with some stuff related to the ex, and it really helped.

I will tell you that it doesn't solve everything. Even a year later, I still get a twinge or two, but the ceremony of burning all of those thoughts and emotions represented a clear turning point for me. It is an important step, and I know from my own experience that it can help you relieve your attachment.

Write about everything. Write about hearing the doctor's words. Write about how you felt as you had to tell people. Write about how you felt as you looked stuff up on the internet. Just let all of those emotions flow out of you. Don't pause to edit anything. Write it out longhand. You're giving yourself permission to feel all of those things.

Remember, as you write all of these words, that none of these things has any power over you any more. They are thoughts, and thoughts have no power unless we take action to make them real.

When you've written everything down, take a few minutes to say goodbye to them. Even though a lot of those thoughts and emotions were negative, they were still your partners and companions over the past several months. You need to get to a place where you can separate them from who you are now and leave them behind.

Only then do you take them over to the fireplace (make sure the flue is open) and light a fire. As it burns, recognize how the smoke dissipates quickly, and the paper turns to ash. There is no structure, no power over you any more.

Be aware that after the ceremony, those emotions and thoughts will come back. They are, after all, a part of what makes you you. But they are a part of your past, and your past cannot hurt you. You've taken away their power.

The Buddhists have a saying, which I'm only now starting to appreciate after both the Tattoo Insight and its Corollary. I look at the world completely differently now, but my position in it hasn't changed. The way they say it is probably something you've come across before: "Before Enlightenment, chop wood and carry water. After Enlightenment, chop wood and carry water."

The world you live in will not be altered dramatically by this ceremony. You'll still be chopping wood and carrying water.

But your perception of it will. And that is everything.

It doesn't happen immediately, but over a surprisingly short period of time you'll find that you are no longer held hostage by those thoughts and emotions, and when it feels like they are taking over, you can remember when you eliminated them from your life. If that isn't enough, you can walk to the fireplace and see their remains in some random ashes.

I performed my ceremony by myself, and it was enormously powerful because I felt like I and I alone was taking control of my life. That was important to me and matched the way that I've gone through life. You may want to do the same. If you want a witness, though, I'd be honored to be there. You just tell me when.

Soon enough, you will understand "There! It's out" in a way that I can't explain via the written word.

Keep adapting. Keep improvising. Keep overcoming.

I love you more than you can possibly imagine.

7/26/12 - Crowdsourcing Inspiration

I've had a Twitter account for years but only use it mainly to rant at companies for bad customer service. At the same time, I use it to follow interesting trends, and one of the most interesting in the past 12 months is the Occupy Wall Street Thing. One of the results of following the Occupy movement is that I came across the Twitter account of a woman named Xeni Jardin. According to her Wikipedia page, she's apparently heavily involved in social media.

I happened to be randomly browsing through Twitter several months ago, and I came across Xeni's live-tweeting of her first mammogram at the age of 41, after which she was diagnosed with breast cancer. She's occasionally funny, sometimes profane, and shows an aptitude for distilling her emotions into 140 characters or less.

Her order of treatment was surgery, then chemo, then radiation. The radiation started yesterday. This was one of her tweets:

@xeni: "Some days I think about cancer more than others. Today, first radiation, I thought a lot. Inspiring words? I got nothin. Cancer just sucks."

She has a ton of followers, one of whom replied with this:

@nickdawson: @xeni patient told me recently: "I just want a day off from cancer, one day when I don't have to think about it".

I know that this isn't necessarily inspirational, except to the extent that you know that there are others who are doing what you're doing. I've read a lot of her tweets - you two seem to me to be kindred spirits at some level. She's in a different place than you right now, as she is just starting radiation, but I see a lot of you in her. If you're looking for something to do, you could do worse than reading her Twitter feed.

In the category of "way more pertinent to your current outlook than the rest of this email", I give you this, which was originally retweeted by a Steelers Blogger that I follow:

@Alexis_Green10: "Stop being afraid of what could go wrong, and start being positive about what could go right."

I looked a little deeper at her profile, mainly because I'm a guy, and her picture showed blond hair. Yes, you should definitely judge me. But here's what I found, in part:

"Alexis. 18. Going to GWU. God is Love." I excluded the rest of the profile because it is representative of the thought processes of an 18 year old blond chick.

Help and inspiration come from the most unusual of places; don't discount the message because of the source. Thomas Jefferson, the greatest advocate of liberty and freedom that the world has ever seen, did so while he literally owned people.

But at the end of the day, God IS love. We're bathing in it, every day, and we don't see it. That's the real tragedy.

I know that this transition isn't going to happen overnight, but I want to repeat something:

"Stop being afraid of what could go wrong, and start being positive about what could go right."

You are on the right path. You're doing all of the right things. Every test says so. It is time for you to Believe. Send the negative thoughts away. Their time is through.

I'm not so optimistic as to suggest that this is going to happen today, or even to say that it should happen within a given time period. It will happen on its own schedule and in its own time. You can't force it, but it will happen.

Remember that thoughts have no power over you, that they disappear like a fart in the wind. Choose your own path, just as your soul did before you were born.

Keep adapting. Keep improvising. Keep overcoming.

I love you more than you can possibly imagine, even though you have ditched your JesusPhone for an imperfect copy. We will be talking about that decision at great length, and when you recognize the error of your ways, I'm going to claim my ApplePoints when we jump you back into the cult.

Text Messages: 7/27/12 5:23 PM

Me: You're halfway to home. I'll be beside you every step of the way, no matter what you need.

Carla: Thank you!

Me: You're welcome. Keep healing!

Me: Believe that you can do it.

Carla: What r you doing?

Me: Watching the Olympic opening ceremony and judging openly. You?

Carla: Same.

Me: Ridiculous doesn't even start to cover it.

Me: I love you. I want you to know that you are going to win. Keep that it your heart. Know it and believe it.

Carla: I told you Phelps should have stayed home. 14 is enough. Time for others to shine

Me: Too many bong hits in the intervening 4 years.

Carla: No, just not knowing when enough is enough. It's like all those boomers who refuse to step aside for another generation.

7/28/12 - Pursuit

I haven't forgotten about you. I saw your texts and I knew you were ready to engage. I'm really sorry that I couldn't tonight. It was really important that I bonded with OLM people so that I would be in a position to support you going forward.

In essence - one step back, three steps forward. The net effect is that a) all of OLM is behind you, and b) I have the freedom to be wherever I need to be, whenever I need to be. Yes, tequila was involved. I play to win, and I am not above cheating to get what I want. Judge as much as you feel is necessary.

I can do these things because I know that you are healing. I know that in 6 weeks you will be free to pursue your life and to learn what your soul chose for you before you were born.

Jefferson's insanely simple Mission Statement seems appropriate:

We hold these truths to be self-evident, that all men are created equal, that they are endowed by their Creator with certain unalienable Rights, that among these are Life, Liberty and the pursuit of Happiness.

You are really close to pursuing Happiness. What form will it take?

Keep adapting. Keep improvising. Keep overcoming.

I love you more than you can possibly imagine. Keep being who you are.

Text Messages: 7/29/12 3:38 PM

Carla: Big day. Went to brunch and then went to Target. Nap time.

Me: Love it. Keep healing!!!

Me: Hope you're doing well today. See you tomorrow.

Carla: Doing ok. I'm at my goal weight as of today so that is a good thing. Just taking it easy today and getting ready for tomorrow. See u then.

7/29/12 - Samothrace

If, like me, you see signs on a regular basis, and you believe that there are no coincidences, this may have some meaning for you.

Inside the stall at Molly McGuire's in Ballard, I noticed a couple of weeks ago, that there is a single word carved into the wood: Samothrace.

After seeing this word, again and again, and again, I decided to do a little digging - why would a Greek word show up in the bathroom of an Irish bar?

Samothrace is a Greek island, but it is better known for a statue that was found there in 1863 - The Winged Goddess of Victory. It now resides at the Louvre as part of its permanent collection.

I read the Wikipedia description. A couple of sentences that apply directly to you stood out:

"The work is notable for its convincing rendering of a pose where violent motion and sudden stillness meet." We've talked at length about the reality that chemo symptoms are going to show up regardless of your mental state. The above statement seems to capture that concept really well.

The full name of the statue is actually The Nike of Samothrace (yes, Nike stole that concept - it means victory - here's to ancient intellectual property!)

Anyway, further down the Wikipedia definition, something stood out: "Nike of Samothrace is seen as an iconic depiction of triumphant spirit and of the divine momentarily coming face to face with man."

I freely admit that I'm still figuring out this whole God thing, and I how I fit into it. I know enough to know that I know next to nothing. But I like that description of "the divine momentarily coming to face with man." It is transcendent. It is, (once again, too much about me and not enough about you), what I've been searching for for a very long time.

I don't know what any of this means for you. Maybe it is as simple as the fact that I keep seeing something that translates to Victory for you. Maybe it is something deeper. Maybe there are NO coincidences.

You're halfway home, Carla. There is nothing easy about the path that you are following, but you can see the path out of the woods now. When you get out of the woods, I know that you want to travel. I understand that it isn't easy to travel long distances, but if you find France on your itinerary, you could do a lot worse than a visit to The Winged Goddess of Victory.

Keep adapting. Keep improvising. Keep overcoming.

I love you more than you can possibly imagine.

7/30/12 - Empty

I want you to know that I believe in you. I want you to know that while I cannot possibly understand what you've endured, I am in absolute awe that you have. I also want you to know what I do, down to the core of my being - your efforts are not in vain. You will survive; more than that, you're going to thrive.

It is a common practice for swimmers to wear extra clothes or weights while training so that they are that much stronger and lighter on race days. You're soon going to shed those clothes and weights that have been holding you back for the past 7 months.

I've asked the question before, but what are your plans for the life you live after the life you learn with? You've earned the right to do nothing, but that isn't you. Doing nothing with what you've learned is as likely as me giving up Sudoku puzzles.

Keep improvising. Keep adapting. Keep overcoming.

I love you more than you can imagine.

7/31/12 - Random thoughts

- As I said in the text on Tuesday night, thank you so much for choosing me to be your pickup person. It means so much to me to be able to do this for you that I can't express it properly. I'm really proud to fill this role for you.

- I really think you came to the right conclusion on what the temporary nurse said - she has no knowledge of what is actually going on. You can confirm that with The Naturopath on Thursday. At the same time, you should probably discuss the circumstances of what she said, and who she said it in front of, with the head nurse. There's never any reason to accept mediocrity.

- I don't know how to say this politely, so I won't. If you don't stop talking about gaining too much weight, I will bury you alive in a box. Stop It. I saw you at 112, and it scared the living crap out of me. Right now, weight gives you space and time, and that's all you need to win this fight. Keep eating like a teenaged boy.

- You can always lose that weight. If necessary, I'll do the PT with you. I'm not fucking around about this. I've gone through it, and I've discovered one truth about PT: The Pain Will End. It will start up 24 hours later, but the pain only lasts for 30 minutes, and after what you've been through, that's not even a light workout. You have the mental training to get through it and to thrive. The best part is that unlike the physical battles that you've gone through over the last 7 months, PT actually MAKES YOU STRONGER.

- I can't really describe the sense of accomplishment that you will feel, of finally taking control of your own destiny for the first time in a very long time. This is the Pursuit of Happiness at its finest.

- Yes, I know that I'm beating a dead horse with this next part. I don't care. It is that important. The first several weeks, maybe even the first month, will suck. You'll feel weak and inadequate and awkward. That's normal. But it does get better. I know this for a fact. I've lived it.

- Do not let the weakness or the awkwardness get you down. You will get stronger and more capable. Unlike your experience with chemo and its side effects, you can be assured that you will prevail.

- Whatever happens with the PT, do not stop. If you need a partner, I'm there. Take control of your destiny, no matter how much it hurts, and no matter how much you want to quit.

Because if you quit, I will bury you alive in a box. You are better than that. You deserve to feel the satisfaction that comes after a PT session, when you are sweaty and shaky and, most important, you've taken control of your own life.

I'm really looking forward to seeing you on Thursday, and as I said at the beginning, I can't thank you enough for picking me to be the pickup guy on Tuesdays. It means more to me than you could possibly imagine.

August

Text Messages: 8/1/12 7:30 PM

Me: Still walking around with a huge grin on my face. 6.9!!!!!!!!

Carla: Me too!

Me: Ok, I'm going to say it again, just to make it really really. Six point FUCKING nine.

Me: Congratulations. Keep kicking ass. You are my hero.

8/1/12 - Letter to Family / Friends

It has been a while since the last update, and the good news keeps rolling in. I picked Carla up from chemo yesterday, and all of her test results, while a little out of the normal range, are exactly what the docs were hoping for.

There is a final test that they do which takes a day or so to run - the cancer marker test. She maxed out at 11 six weeks ago, then dropped to a 9.5 two weeks ago. I'm not sure of the scale, other than that lower is better, but The Naturopath assured us that it was all positive.

Carla called me this afternoon and asked me if I was sitting down, because the number had just come in. I'd been dreading this all day, but there was something in her voice that told me that this was a good kind of sitting down request.

Today's result: 6.9 (anything below 5 is considered cancer-free).

To say that she's ecstatic understates things quite a bit. Finally, everything she has been doing is paying off. She's found a way to manage the symptoms to the point where she's now at 132 pounds (up from 112) and accepting good-natured ribbing from the nurses about being portly.

A good day all around - I'll keep all updated as events warrant.

8/1/12 - 6.9. Fuck and Yes

The Naturopath asks me, on a regular basis, "what is the story of your life?"

We all have the same basic story - we are born, we do some stuff, and then we die. That's a harsh assessment, but it is true. If the insights that I've had in the last month are true, the do some stuff part is important.

The question I want to ask you is this: what is the life you are going to live after the life that you've learned with? How are you going to convert what you've learned into something that is valuable for the world, and not just for you? You owe the world nothing, but at the same time, I know you. It is in your nature to spread the word.

From Bull Durham -

Annie Savoy: The world is made for people who aren't cursed with self awareness.

How do we move forward in a world where self awareness is not a prized trait?

After my Tattoo Insight, and the subsequent corollary, I'm struck by the number of people walking around who don't get this basic concept. I don't do it in a mean-spirited way, or in a judgmental way (for once) - we all proceed at our own pace.

Time for our Wall Street interlude -

Bud Fox: Sun-tzu - If your enemy is superior, evade him. If angry, irritate him. If equally matched, fight, and if not split and reevaluate.

Lou Mannheim: Man looks in the abyss, there's nothing staring back at him. At that moment, man finds his character. And that is what keeps him out of the abyss.

You have stared into the abyss, and you stayed out of it. You've evaded your enemy, you've irritated him, and in the end, you are going to defeat him. I could not be happier or prouder of you than I am now. There is only one thing left to do in a world where The Simpsons exists.

Mr. Burns: Smithers, release the hounds.

Don't give your enemy a chance to rest. You have the advantage now. Use every dirty trick in the book.

Blue Horseshoe loves Annacot Steel.

Keep up the skeer.

Keep improvising. Keep adapting. Keep overcoming.

I love you more than you can possibly imagine.

Text Messages: 8/4/12 5:16 PM

Me: From Brad - "Saw the comment from your mom. Katie and I are toasting to Carla and cheering for her full recovery and to having a long healthy life filled with cocaine addition."

Carla: Love it!

8/4/12 - The Story

I'd like to think that I've become more sensitive to the ripples in the pond that is life because of a lot of stuff that has gone on, not just with you, but from my perspective in general.

Last Saturday, I went to a wedding reception for my coworker Nikol. She has turned out to be an absolute find, and she will be a long term asset to OLM if we have the wit to let her grow beyond her currently defined role. It isn't difficult to spot the ones who get it, and she is one of those.

Anyway, she's also apparently a backup singer for a local band. Don't ask me the name. These things escape me. The band played her reception, and Nikol got one solo - she did "The Story" by Brandi Carlile, and absolutely nailed it.

In the days since, I keep listening to this song. It is just so powerful, so full of raw emotion. Disregard the words, which are lonely and plaintive, asking for someone to share her story. Or don't disregard them. The sharing of stories is what makes us human.

Remember the introduction to Amazing Stories, with a wizened old guy sitting around a campfire? We are genetically built for this type of thing. The Naturopath 's insistence on the fact that we need to write our own story lives at the intersection of genetics and spirituality.

It sounds like you started to rewrite your story on Thursday. Where will it lead?

For inspiration, here's video of The Story performed live. Crank it up and let the emotion flow through you. All things are possible.

http://www.youtube.com/watch?v=o8pQLtHTPaI&sns=e
m

Keep improvising. Keep adapting. Keep overcoming.

I love you more than you can possibly imagine, and I can't thank you enough for letting me in to your life.

8/4/12 - The Clean Slate

Do you remember buying the Spiderman 2 game for PS2? I'm reasonably certain that you did not play it the whole way through. I did.

Once you have beaten the final villain, the narrator comes on and says something like "welcome to the rest of your life - you're going to spend it rescuing little old ladies from muggers."

The point is, even if you have superpowers, the Buddhist statement remains: "Before Enlightenment, chop wood and carry water. After Enlightenment, chop wood and carry water."

You have reached a point where you can start to put cancer in your rear view mirror (this would have a lot more impact if you actually drove, but one step at a time. I think it is time for you to learn how to drive, as long as there is no risk of me blowing up in the driveway).

At any rate, it is time to start writing your story. I know that you are champing at the bit to move forward. Channel that energy into planning and plotting how you will return.

I know that this is not satisfying right now. It will pay huge dividends.

But don't just plot your return. Plot your ascendancy. Be better than you ever thought you could be. Do things that you've never imagined.

Every single thing is possible for you. There are no restrictions. This is the time to write your own ticket, to slay the dragons of stupidity that you've had to compromise with for the last decade. Do not lose this opportunity.

You are easily one of the most brilliant people I've ever known, and your ability to translate brilliance into results is well-documented.

What are you waiting for? Get ready to take the world by storm. You are one of the few on this planet who can do so.

Keep adapting. Keep improvising. Keep overcoming.

I love you more than you can possibly imagine.

8/5/12 - The Grind

A lot of professional golfers talk about grinding out on the course. To them, it means hitting fairways and greens and two-putting and accepting pars, because the risks that are involved with putting yourself in position to score birdies and eagles are far too high in comparison to the reward.

It means doing what is necessary and accepting the boring outcome, and above all, being patient. Courses are set up to reward the patient, with some holes, especially on the back nine, set up to reward the bold and the skillful. But up until about the twelfth hole, the courses are set up to reward those who can stay patient and grind it out.

Right now you're in the midst of a set of holes that are boring and set up in such a way that the best way to play is to grind it out. To take your pars. To be patient.

It isn't a lot of fun, and it is a little stressful. There aren't birdies and eagles available to make your efforts feel like they are having some impact.

But those pars add up after a while. You keep grinding for long enough, and those birdie opportunities will present themselves. Like last Wednesday, when 6.9 presented itself.

You are doing everything right. You're making pars when you need to, and your score reflects that fact. Keep patient and keep grinding. What you are doing now is incredibly important.

I love you more than you can possibly imagine.

Text Messages: 8/7/12 9:33 PM

Carla: Thank you again for staying. That was a bit rough last night so thanks for being here.

Me: It is my honor to be asked and to be trusted to help during a difficult time. Keep healing.

Carla: Well that was a bit rougher than normal. The side effects change from round to round so i never know what to expect from week to week.

Me: I know. I think we've managed to find something that doesn't work, and I'll keep that in mind in the future.

Carla: Its late and a school night. Shouldnt you be getting home?

Me: Still doing my homework. I have a composition to write.

Carla: Yes you do. And may i just say your intended audience is a bit shaky this evening and could use a bit of help. No pressure.

Me: That actually makes it easier, now that I know what to talk about.

Me: Carla, sooner than you know you will be living a cancer free life. This experience will always be with you, but it will not dominate your destiny, and it will not define who you are.

8/7/12 - Winning 20 in the Show

About a million years ago, in the summer of 2000, John and Tom and I got into an argument about the email communications that they were sending out to customers. As you know, I am a bit of a grammar and spelling Nazi, and they were sending out these typo-filled nightmares that reflected so badly on the company that I banned them from sending anything out for 6 months without me proofreading it.

When they objected, I needed to quote only one movie (Bull Durham) for them to understand how important this was:

Crash Davis: "Your shower shoes have fungus on them. You'll never make it to the bigs with fungus on your shower shoes. Think classy, you'll be classy. If you win 20 in the show, you can let the fungus grow back and the press'll think you're colorful. Until you win 20 in the show, however, it means you are a slob."

Let me be clear on something, as we both know that you could not even come close to my level of slovenliness. That's not what I'm talking about here. I'm talking about confidence and belief and feeling Grace in your life.

Has 6.9 taught you nothing? Has gaining weight DURING chemo taught you nothing? Has being named the ideal patient taught you nothing? You are healing.

You have endured the unendurable. Look at the things that you've done. Do you honestly think you could have done these things unless you are stronger than you thought you were?

You are not going to fail. Every single indicator tells us this, and don't discount The Naturopath's understanding

330

of your pulses. It is weird and subjective, but if he isn't feeling anything bad going on, trust him. There is a reason that you met him. Trust what he told you, that you are ready to move to the next part of your life, free from this scourge.

You do not have fungus on your metaphorical shower shoes, and even when you win 20 games in The Show, you still won't need to rely on your shower shoes to convince the world that you're colorful and have something to offer.

More important than that, remember the lesson that we've talked about so many times - if you want to be an actor, then BE an actor.

Getting to "There, It's Out" can sometimes seem to be an impossible task. You are really close, and sometimes the only thing it takes is to understand that the only difference between knowing the path and walking the path is the distinctions and walls that we build for ourselves.

There are no limits on what we can do. There are only limits on what we allow ourselves to do. Believe in the process. Believe in yourself.

I believe in you, because my belief has been tested, and my faith rewarded. Trust in the Grace that flows through your life.

Keep improvising. Keep adapting. Keep overcoming.

I love you more than you can possibly imagine. Keep healing.

8/8/12 - Noise in the neurons

I've been thinking quite a bit about you today as I've gone through my day and reread some of the emails I've sent you. As you know, I do this mainly to remind myself of the things that I've said, but also because I have been picking up on some trends and themes.

I've decided that if I ever do end up publishing these things, I'm going to do it strictly as an e-book. The first half of the book will be the emails organized by date, because it is interesting to see the ebbs and flows. When all of this started I had no idea what to expect or what to do or how to help. Maybe this grouping will help someone who is caring for another to understand the ebbs and flows.

The second half will be the same letters, but organized into some sort of thematic grouping. If you're interested, once I get things organized, I'm hoping you might do either a little foreword or afterword on each of these groups. This is more for the person who is actually going through it. The letters are short enough that you can pick one up randomly, and depending on the section, maybe it helps to get that person through a difficult night.

It is against this backdrop that I recognize that although we've touched on it, we have focused a lot on healing your body, but very little on healing your soul and spirit.

There is no way for you to come away from this without being irrevocably touched and altered. But just like your body has proven incredibly resilient against this disease, and the nearly-as-bad treatments, your spirit and your soul are just as strong, if not stronger.

We've only talked a little about how you are doing in your emotional recovery from what was a truly devastating time in your life, and what I perceive as your continuing worry about "what if". I'm not nearly naive enough to say that these feelings will fade, or the emotions and worry you've attached to them are any less real than your physical struggle.

I guess the only thing I would try to remind you is that these are only thoughts. Strong and upsetting ones, to be sure, but only thoughts. They have, at the end of the day, no power over you.

The strength of your mind and your spirit and your soul have sustained you for 8 long months. You only got through it because of who you are. Now your body is healing, and it is time to reverse the flows.

Take emotional strength from the amazing rebound that your body has made. Take spiritual strength from how strong you remain in the face of all you have endured. Use your time with the physical therapist to rebuild your confidence as you rebuild your body.

Above all, never doubt that you will be well again, and a lot sooner than you think. You don't have to fight negative thoughts to beat them. You just have to recognize that there is no need to fight them - they are nothing but what Cryptonomicon calls noise in the neurons.

Keep improvising. Keep adapting. Keep overcoming.

I love you more than you can possibly imagine.

Text Messages: 8/9/12 9:14 PM

Carla: I think the title of noise in the neurons is my favorite one so far.

Me: I'm glad you liked it. I got it from Neal Stephenson and really think that it distilled the concept so well.

8/9/12 - The egg

This one is going to be short. For once.

A couple of thoughts, both sports-related. I am who I am.

Crash Davis in Bull Durham: "This game's fun, OK? Fun, Goddammit! And don't hold the ball so hard, OK? It is an egg. Hold it like an egg!"

The second one is something that I read while learning to play golf back when I was 8 - I don't have a link, because the advice is about 60 years old, way before Al Gore invented the Internet -"hold the club as if it were a bird - too much pressure and you kill the bird; not enough, and the bird will fly away."

You're smart enough to figure out how this applies to you. Anything else is just noise in the neurons.

Keep improvising. Keep adapting. Keep overcoming.

I love you more than you can possibly imagine.

Text Messages: 8/10/12 5:21 PM

Carla: Now im camped in the parking lof of a walmart. I am about 15 yrs too young for this lifestyle.

Me: Think of it as an adventure.

Carla: That is exactly what this is. Im lovin every minute of it.

Me: I'm thrilled that you're doing this. Good for you.

Carla: So far so goo. We are having fun.

Text Messages: 8/12/12 6:22 PM

Carla: Thank god for drugs and big bang theory. 3 hours tonight.

Me: Whatever it takes.

Carla: Oh this show relaxes me and takes my mind off everything. I could watch it all day.

Me: I know. Plus it is funny, has some heart and soul to it, and you can learn something from it.

Carla: Its perfect.

8/14/12 - The most difficult discipline

(I bought Carla a couple of books to keep her entertained and motivated. Both of them occupy a unique place in my psyche.)

Both of the books have special meaning for me, and I gave you both of them for very specific reasons. I want you to understand why, and I want you to understand how they speak to you more eloquently than I ever possibly could.

Harold And The Purple Crayon defined my first year or two at OLM - when you read the book, you'll see the parallels. Whenever Harold gets into a predicament, he is able to draw his way out of it, like when he is flailing around in the water - he gets out of it by drawing a boat. OLM was so new that we could get away with making stuff up as we went along.

It was only years later, in consultation with The Naturopath and his repeating theme - we are all writing our own stories - that I realized that there is a larger lesson from this very simple book that I had only seen as a metaphor for how we built OLM.

It doesn't matter where we are in the cycle. We can always begin again. Most importantly, we are always able to take control and write our own story. It only takes the understanding that we control the purple crayon.

A Wish For Wings That Work is a slightly different animal. I pull it out every couple of months, usually when I'm feeling down about where I am in my life, and when I am questioning how I fit in.

Sometimes that second question is debilitating. It certainly was this weekend after the Danielle Debacle. I can't really explain how difficult it is to live on the far fringes, seemingly always a spectator, always yearning, but ultimately resigned to the fact that, as Obi-Wan said, my "destiny lies along a different path," when that path is ill-defined and rarely taken.

Oh, like you thought you were going to escape this without a Star Wars quote.

But the truth that I want you to understand is that we all have wings that work. Sometimes that takes a different form than what we expect, and it is up to us to be patient enough to let it develop.

Patience is the hardest discipline of all. But it has the greatest rewards. We just have to have our purple crayon ready to write our story. Is your purple crayon nearby?

I've asked you the question enough times - what are you going to do with the life you live after you've lived the life you've learned with? Are you patient enough, as Dex says in The Tao of Steve, to be desireless, to be excellent, and to be gone with respect to your larger purpose? You don't owe anybody anything, and shutting down is an option; I think I know you well enough that it isn't an option for you.

Keep improvising. Keep adapting. Keep overcoming.

I love you more than you can possibly imagine.

8/16/12 - Throw the slider

I've been thinking quite a bit about all the things that you've had to go through and all that you've accomplished. I think I may have found a reasonable metaphor for you to think about in terms of Felix Hernandez's perfect game.

There have been 23 perfect games in baseball history. In a lot of them, there is some luck involved. About 25% of the pitchers who have one went on to toil in obscurity with one magical day as their high point.

By and large, however, perfect games are thrown by pitchers at the top of their games. Their stuff is, to use a word, filthy. It is almost like they are playing against a high school team.

But it is more than raw dominance of one specific pitch that makes for a perfect game. It is the ability to switch tactics seamlessly and to be able to both throw conventional pitches in conventional situations and to throw, with confidence, pitches that make no sense in context of the game situation or the count.

The best example of this from yesterday came in the ninth inning. Felix Hernandez threw two balls to the second batter. A situation like this normally calls for a fastball, something that will absolutely be called for a strike. The danger of this approach is that the hitter knows this as well - he is waiting for the fastball.

John Jaso, the catcher, also knew this, so he called for a slider. This is one of the most difficult pitches to throw, but when it is on, it is effectively unhittable. This one went for a strike, the next pitch, an equally unhittable curve ball, went for a strike, and on an even count, Felix induced the hitter into a weak ground ball for an easy out.

Why all of this baseball theory? Because given everything you've had to face, you've had to do almost everything perfectly. You've had to have command of four or five different pitches. You've had to be able to switch between tactics seamlessly. And you needed a catcher (in my mind, this is The Naturopath) willing to tell you to throw the slider in a 2-0 count because he knows you can deliver.

The more I think about it, the more this metaphor works. Even the number of months parallels the length of a baseball game.

So here we are. You're in the top of the ninth. You have a perfect game going, and your catcher wants you to throw the slider.

You have it in your arsenal.

You have been displaying your adaptability for nearly 9 months.

Throw the slider.

I love you more than you can possibly imagine.

8/16/12 - Letter to Family / Friends

I'll keep this one short. Since the cancer marker tests began, Carla has had a 12, 14, 11, 9.5, and a 6.9

This week's number: 5.6

She feels like crap, but that's the chemo, not her getting worse. We're in the middle of round 6, with two more to go. After that is a single CT test on 9/21, and then she's clear.

Her docs are all unanimous that she's doing great and are even going to limit the CT scan to her abdomen only, rather than checking her chest and brain.

These are much better times. Even she is starting to believe it, and she and Stu are beginning the planning for their first celebratory road trip, to see the Redwoods and Yosemite, which they're going to do in early October.

Thanks to all who've let me work through some of this via overly long, rambling, ranting emails.

Text Messages: 8/29/12 5:52 PM

Me: 4.4 - still can't believe it. I'm so happy for you.

Carla: I feel the same way.

Carla: Thank you again so much for helping me get through it.

Me: You're welcome. It has been an honor to play a role. Now we just have to get you through the next 21 days.

Me: You're doing great. Your resolve to see this all the way through is inspiring.

Carla: I hope this news inspires you as i have not received an email in quite sometime. I re-read past ones for a lift.

Me: Blame that on the job. It has drained me, and my muse has not visited in a long time. I really can't describe what writing those things is like - there is zero effort, and it flows out with zero direction from me.

Me: I have started and deleted over a dozen emails, because they were just terrible and forced and you deserve the very best.

Me: I'm going to vote for a Democrat for president. That is how much both of them piss me off.

Carla: I hear ya. Most depressing election of my lifetime.

8/29/12 - Letter to Family / Friends

With one month left (she's in the middle of round 7 of chemo), it is time for the reveal of the cancer marker number. Since the cancer marker tests began, Carla has had a 12, 14, 11, 9.5, 7.9, and a 5.6.

Today's number is 4.4 - she's effectively cancer-free, but has made the decision with her docs to finish all 8 rounds despite the fact that the deeper she gets into this the more the side effects are starting to pile up. In her case, it is low blood pressure and anemia that are the main foes right now, as well as some lingering pain.

21 days of hell left.

September

Text Messages: 9/2/12 5:02 PM

Carla: Good to hear that the project is going well. Im okay just so so tired.

Me: I know you are. It will end soon.

Carla: Don't say it like that;-) It will be all better soon!

Me: You know what I meant. All of the crap you've been dealing with will end soon and you will return to full health.

Carla: Keep thinking that. Everyday just a bit closer.

Carla: At times I feel strong and at times just feel overwhelmed by everything that I have been through these past nine months. Today I am tired and emotional.

Me: Being emotional is to be expected. What you have done is incredible.

Me: You're welcome for the email. It was nice to be able to finally tell you all of those things.

Carla: Thank you for all of your kind words and support. I could not have done this without you.

Me: I'm happy that I could help in whatever way possible. I'm even happier that you've found a way through.

Carla: I need to find that meaning and new life.

Me: You will. Just walk the path. If you go searching for it, you'll never find it. Live your life, but be aware.

Me: Always, though, you will know that nothing can ever scare you again. You may not have conquered fear, but you have stared it down.

9/2/12 - Charts

I haven't written a lot lately. A lot of this is because, quite frankly, I've felt that you are out of the danger zone for a while. As you once said, my output is directly proportional to my stress level. I look back at the things that I've said and written, and I can almost chart my stress level based on the things that I wrote.

But I want to talk, hopefully briefly, about a different kind of chart. I've been tracking your CEA numbers ever since they started coming out. Every other Wednesday is an exercise in self control to not call you at 3 in the afternoon.

I love that you preface it all, every time, with "are you sitting down", and then spend 5 minutes talking about everything other than what we really want to talk about. I love that the first huge drop was delivered while I was sitting on my back porch and I think I offended every neighbor within 5 blocks by saying "are you fucking kidding me?" again and again.

Because I am who I am, I've kept a graph of that number open on my PC. This week, I printed it out. It faces me, so that whenever I look up, I see it. It is right beside my whiteboard, upon which is written three of my favorite axioms:

- Know your enemy and be faster than him (Saddam Hussein)
- The enemy of the good is the pefect (Phil Condit)
- EMBRACE AMBIGUITY (uncredited)

Each of these things reminds me of something important.

- The Saddam quote - even crazy people are right from time to time.
- Look closely at the Condit quote. Notice anything spelled wrong? That's the point.
- UNCREDITED is me telling myself to accept gray areas.

I look at these things every single day. I added a graph of your CEA numbers to the cork board.

This is not done to remind me to call you.

This is done to remind me that (pardon the caps) EVERYTHING IS POSSIBLE. When I feel low, I look at that graph, and I think about what you did to make it possible, and I am in awe.

For once, words are failing me. I'm trying to figure out how to tell you how much I respect you, how much, quite frankly, you are an inspiration to me.

I know that, in the words of Robert Frost, you have miles to go before you can rest easy. Hard doesn't even come close to describing it.

I guess I just wanted you to know how much your strength and your resilience has affected me and, quite frankly, improved me.

Ray Kinsella: "It was you..."

Shoeless Joe: "No, Ray, it was you..."

You've had this in you all along, Carla. What you've done is a testament to who you are.

Like the dog in The Art of Racing In The Rain, all I have is large gestures. All I can do is to say thank you, and that doesn't even come close to the right expression of my respect, my admiration, my thanks for everything.

You are unique and special and dynamic and about nine other adjectives, and I am privileged to call you my friend.

I love you, more than you will ever know. Keep adapting. Keep improvising. Keep overcoming

9/3/12 - Odds

You once told me that the thing you respected about me the most is that I didn't really seem to care too much about what others thought of me.

Now let me tell you what I respect most about you. Surprisingly enough, it has very little to do with the last 9 months. Ok, it has a little to do with it, but it is something I saw in you back in 1999.

I remember you being completely freaked out in the summer of 1999 about the prospect of having to do an introductory speech in front of 100 people.

A week later, you did it, and nobody ever knew what you were experiencing. You know why? It isn't that you have no fear. It is that you refuse to allow it to dominate you. You face fear better than anyone I know, and as someone who is afraid to even try a different hamburger, or, indeed, to put ketchup on my hot dogs, let alone try the plethora of ethnic foods available in our amazing city, you are a model that I can only hope to live up to some day.

I can't imagine how scared you've been on a regular basis for the past 9 months. But here is the important part - you kept doing what needed to be done. You showed up. You walked the hallway. You never backed down.

You're about to graduate from the hardest school on earth. You've made chemo your ally, not your enemy, by realizing that chemo is part of your team. You've beaten the odds, in large part, I believe, because there is a bit of Han Solo in you.

C-3PO: Sir, the chances of successfully navigating an asteroid field is approximately 3,720 to 1

Han Solo: Never tell me the odds!

I love you more than you can possibly imagine. Keep adapting. Keep improvising. Keep overcoming.

9/5/12 - The end of fear

I've been thinking a lot about the next part of your life. I know that you, for lots of reasons, all of them pretty good, (mainly, getting through the next 15 days), don't want to spend a lot of time thinking about this.

If you're really serious about keeping that mindset, not a problem. Save this one for later. It can keep, because it is about the lessons that all of us should already know, and which we keep relearning, again and again.

If you're back, or if you are just curious, hi.

Foxism: If you don't go, you'll never know. If you don't try, you'll never know why.

Foxism: At least a billion people have done this before you.

You know what these two Foxisms are about? Fear. Fear of the unknown. Fear of looking foolish. Fear of being hurt. Fear of being afraid.

These are not fears that should worry you any more. You've put your fear to the side. You've walked with it. Look at the stuff that you've done. You could not have done it if you were the type of person who succumbs to fear. You've conquered the unknown. You've conquered being hurt.

Let's just go ahead and get Biblical:

The Lord is my Shepherd; I shall not want.
He maketh me to lie down in green pastures:
He leadeth me beside the still waters.
He restoreth my soul:

He leadeth me in the paths of righteousness for His name'
sake.

Yea, though I walk through the valley of the shadow of
death,
I will fear no evil: For thou art with me;
Thy rod and thy staff, they comfort me.
Thou preparest a table before me in the presence of mine
enemies;
Thou annointest my head with oil; My cup runneth over.

Surely goodness and mercy shall follow me all the days of
my life,
and I will dwell in the House of the Lord forever.

You have walked through the Valley of the Shadow of
Death. You have stared into the abyss. You have nothing
left to fear.

You have some hard days left, I am sure. But you have
already displayed that you have what it takes to do so.

I know that this is simplistic, but I want you to know that
the past 9 months have shown me what I knew all along.

You are easily the strongest person I know. You deserve
this part of the Psalm that I quoted above:

"Surely goodness and mercy shall follow me all the days
of my life."

I love you more than you can possibly imagine. Keep
improvising. Keep adapting. Keep overcoming.

9/7/12 - Next

I look back on the string of emails, and I can only come to one conclusion. You were meant to survive. You've done the impossible.

There is a temptation to say, "ok, what are you going to do with this understanding?"

That is bullshit. Why should you have to do anything special after, in your words, "looking in to the Abyss?". Did the bar for enjoying your life suddenly get raised as a result of being close to the end of it?

No.

You're 14 days away from freedom, from liberty, from being sprung from prison. Live your life on your own terms, not on what any other person expects of you because you've gone through hell.

You've earned the right to do what you want to do. The choices you decide to make are yours, and yours alone. You don't need to validate them with anybody.

I love you more than you can possibly imagine. Keep adapting. Keep improvising. Keep overcoming.

9/8/12 - After

I'm almost certain that as you get close to the end of your treatment, you are getting buried in Shawshank Redemption quotes. If you aren't, let me know, and I will bury you in Shawshank Redemption quotes.

But that is so shallow. It doesn't touch what you've lived through, or what you've accomplished. It doesn't come close to recognizing how hard it was. Part of me doesn't really want to know - it is too much.

I am in awe of what you've done. More than anything, you kept getting up and doing the things that your docs asked of you. It wasn't pleasant. It wasn't easy. But you kept doing it. AND IT FUCKING WORKED.

After 9 long months, you are about to be set free. No more doctors. No more rounds of chemo. No more people dictating a schedule of narcotics. No more people telling you what to do.

Freedom.

Liberty.

I can't begin to imagine how both a) exciting and b) scary this is for you. I want you to know that I will be there with you every step of the way, no matter what it takes. My commitment to you does not end with an all-clear declaration from your docs.

You are my best friend. Whenever you need me, I will be there.

You will recover. You will thrive.

I love you more than you can possibly imagine.

Keep improvising. Keep adapting. Keep overcoming.

Text Messages: 9/9/12 1:17 PM

Me: Miracles do happen. You've seen it. Start drinking the kool-aid.

Carla: Yes I believe I have.

Me: I know. You're amazing. The things that you have done are beyond description.

Me: Keep believing in miracles. They happen every single day. You are a walking example of this.

Carla: Thanks for these encouraging words.

Me: You never backed down. You never gave up an inch. That is encouraging to me.

Carla: I think you give me too much credit.

Me: I don't think I give you enough. When I grow up I want to be you.

Me: You have a set of brass balls that I can only envy.

Carla: I don't know about that. All I do is eat and sleep. No brass balls needed for that.

Carla: Thank you. Thid next week is so critical and I'm trying to be calm and positive.

Me: Stay yourself. Don't worry about being positive. Be who you are. Breathe. BELIEVE.

Me: Just in case you are reading this in the middle of the night -

Me: Believe in who you are. Breathe your amazing nature. In and out.

Me: Know that you are going to put this awful time in your past.

Text Messages: 9/12/12 6:04 PM

Me: Just realized that they pulled the line today. What a nice early birthday present - no more chemo!

Carla: Yes. It was nice to be freed from my longtime friend. I think we are both going ready to moce on.

Me: Exactly. And the best part is that your old friend won't be drunk-texting you in an attempt to get back together.

Text Messages: 9/13/12 7:30 AM

Me: Good morning! Happy Birthday!

Me: Welcome to the first day of the rest of your life. From here on out, it is about healing. No more treatment. No more recovery from visits from your teammate.

Carla: Thank you. I feel wonderful today. Despite chemo effects I am so happy to have come this far. Best birthday ever!

Me: Stay awesome. Keep believing.

Carla: I am. I will. So much to be happy about today. Going to enjoy it.

Me: I am so happy for you.

Text Messages: 9/17/12 10:18 PM

Me: I tried to write something awesome in order to commemorate this week. It didn't come, but it was not for lack of effort.

Me: Here's what I have: Keep Healing. Keep getting better every day. You've escaped the cycle.

Me: Live your life however you choose. You've earned that right.

Me: I love you more than you can possibly imagine

Me: Keep improvising. Keep adapting. Keep overcoming.

Text Messages: 9/18/12 6:51 AM

Carla: Thanks for the works of encouragement. I needd that. Somedays are better than others.

Me: You're welcome. More good days are coming, and the bad days will be fewer and fewer.

Carla: I do believe that. As hard as this has been i do believe good times are ahead.

Text Messages: 9/19/12 9:45 PM

Me: I read the book by the Seal who was on the Bin Laden raid. He said the way he got through Seal training was to focus on getting to the next meal.

Me: You're mostly past that phase now, but good to have in your back pocket just in case you need a little motivation.

Carla: Funny. Thats how Ive been getting from one moment to the next. I too focus on my next meal. No joke.

9/19/12 - What next?

One of my favorite stories from one of Robert Fulghum's books is that Benjamin Franklin was in Paris and was invited to the first demonstration of the hot air balloon. One of the French guys on the trip with him took one look, and in typical French fashion (sorry - I grew up conservative - some biases are impossible to erase) said "eh, what good is it?"

Franklin turned to address his compatriot and said "eh, what good is a newborn baby?"

Never mind how you got here. You are here. The field has been swept clean. You have as many possibilities as the newborn baby that Franklin spoke of.

I've been thinking a lot lately about the CIA guy who spoke at Fast Company a lifetime ago. In retrospect, he was talking about the fragility of life, and the ascendancy of the spirit, and, dare I say it, the audacity of hope. Yes, I cringed on typing that last phase.

Given that the field is wide open, I'd like to propose a possible path for you to pursue. It isn't the only path. Just an option.

Speak.

You are so fucking good at it. You have an amazing story to tell. You and I have talked about work-life balance since we met. Since your ordeal began, we've talked about how things got out of whack and were a contributing factor. Talk about how you were the queen of work-life balance and you ignored your own advice.

Some of this is selfish - I want to see you speak again, to control a room. You're the best I've ever seen at it. But more than that, I see a marketing opportunity for you. You're an expert at this stuff. Not "I know this pretty well." An expert. In complete command of the subject.

I know the type. In my limited field, I am one. And in your area of expertise, you are too.

A couple of speeches in front of the right audiences, and your calendar will be full with consulting gigs. At $200/hour. You are that good.

And when you need to sit down and write the companion book that will land you on Oprah, etc., you have a really good ghostwriter who only needs to be paid in scotch. (Note to the lawyers - for a book this good, the scotch payment should be measured in truckloads).

I know I'm looking beyond the moment. I know that you're still recovering. But I want you to understand that there is a world of opportunity ahead of you.

I have believed in your resilience. I have seen it in person. Your strength is a continuing source of inspiration to me.

Keep getting to the next meal.

I love you more than you can possibly imagine.

Keep improvising. Keep adapting. Keep overcoming.

Text Messages: 9/20/12 5:36 PM

Me: Hope your day today was good. What time is the appointment tomorrow?

Carla: 9:30 tomorrow. Im so anxious

Me: This is the culmination of everything you've done. Tomorrow will be your victory day. Tomorrow will make it all worth it.

Carla: I wont know the results until next wed though.

Me: Then there is nothing to be anxious about tomorrow. Next week will be awesome.

Text Messages: 9/21/12 3:50 PM

Carla: All done for today at least. Stu took me to Ihop afterwards for breakfast and then to one of my favorite thrift stores. Best day so far. So happy to be out amoung the living i cant even tell you. Well for about an hour or so, until I got sick and needed to go home. But it felt great even for a little while to be back in the land of the living!

Me: I'm glad to hear that you're feeling well enough to do that.

Me: Keep resting - better days are just around the corner.

Text Messages: 9/24/12 9:17 PM

Carla: Can u believe the end of that game? And I believe in the power of love and faith. That is what makes a miracle. Thank you for being a part of that miracle.

Me: We've talked about the power of grace. You have had it with you every step of the way, and you accepted it into your life.

Me: You made your own miracle. I cannot possibly describe how happy I am for you.

9/24/12 - Large Gestures

You have adapted. You have improvised. You have overcome.

You have proved that nothing is impossible. Thank you for believing. Thank you for persevering and for showing the rest of us what is possible.

I love you more than you can possibly imagine. I can't really describe how happy I am for you right now. Please thank all of your food providers from Garvey for me. Please thank Stu, for standing by you.

I told you at the beginning that you would have to do this by yourself, but you would never do it alone. I can't tell you how proud I am of you, or what an inspiration you are to me.

For once, words fail me. All I have is large gestures. All I can do is sit on my back deck and thank Heaven that you are safe. I know that there is more to it, but that's my limit right now.

God bless, Carla. I love you and I can't wait to see you soon.

9/24/12 - Letter to Family / Friends

257 days after being diagnosed, and after enduring an existence that I would not wish upon my worst enemy, Carla received the report on her last CT from her doc tonight.

COMPLETELY CLEAR. SHE BEAT IT.

I can't even begin to describe how happy I am for her. For the first time since January, she now believes she has a future. I heard the difference in her voice as she delivered the news.

I can't thank all of you enough for listening to me and providing your love and support. Watching this up close has been incredibly difficult, and I couldn't have been there for her if you weren't there for me.

So thank you all, from the bottom of my heart. Each of you helped to save my best friend's life, and I am eternally grateful.

Text Messages: 9/25/12 9:21 AM

Me: Hope you're doing well this morning. Have you been watching the uproar caused by how bad the refs suck?

Carla: Yes and I remember Super Bowl 40 so everyone can suck it. We won!

October

10/7/12 - An accumulation of random thoughts

- First, I am really sorry that I haven't been able to properly celebrate your healing day / clearance / release from prison. There were things that I had to do at work for this changeover, and I was the only one that could do them. I've been thinking about your success every single day, and I am so proud of you / happy for you that I'm about to explode. At the same time, I know that you understand the obligations that I needed to take care of.

- I want to see you and hang out with you as soon as I can. Listening to your voice is so inspiring to me - you are just full of life and hope and joy. It makes doing what I need to do for work, to help this team that we've put together, so much easier. It gives me energy to push through.

- I've come to realize over the last couple of months just how many people depend on me doing my very best, and in an odd way, I think your ordeal/journey helped me to see it. I had to open up, to be completely there in order to help take care of you. Now that I've seen this way of living, I can't go back, and it impacts the way I look at everything. Mind. Blown.

- The Friday conversation was transformative for me. I love that you sent Stu to see Peter Gabriel, and that you have decided to go to Paris, and that you are actively focused on living your life. We can talk about this in person, but I want you to know that moving forward I am taking my inspiration from that conversation. It basically boils down to the fact that I don't want to look back and regret missed opportunities in 30 years.

- I really think that you ought to let the spider live. Too many karmic implications if you whack him. Worst case, we can take him outside.

- I've had a spider on my front porch who keeps building a web in my path. I keep taking down the web without whacking him. Eventually, he learned to build the web on the side of the porch. Now we are both happy - I don't walk through a spider web every morning, and he doesn't have to rebuild every morning. Plus he's still killing everything that gets close to his web.

- The HR people back in Detroit are reorganizing. Again. This time it seems that they are doing a little more emphasis on rewards and recognition. They will, of course, fuck this up unless they have help. I'm not trying to shove you back into the workforce, but I want you to know that when you're ready, I think I can get you an attentive audience for a consulting gig at a stupidly high rate per hour (they are really good at the stupidly high hourly rate thing for consultants).

- For now, of course, your focus needs to be on resting and healing. I respect that and want you to wait. But you are the best I've ever seen in that area - you get it on a level that very few do. I've watched and listened for over a decade. When you switch into that mode, you're a force of nature. Trust me, I recognize greatness when I see it, and you have it.

- Keep thinking about the book. Your story is inspirational and cautionary and a reminder that the medical industry is both awful and amazing at the same time. Whether you pick me or someone else to help you write it, this is a story that needs to be told.

I really want to thank you for everything - for letting me be there during the difficult times, as well as the good ones. I will admit to missing the visits to The Naturopath and picking you up from chemo, even as I don't miss the reasons why I was doing both things. Speaking selfishly, those trips and staying over were so personal and so...intimate is the wrong word, but I don't have a better one. I want to say thank you for sharing them with me.

You're the best person that I have ever known. I am humbled and honored that you've chosen me as a friend.

I love you more than you can possibly imagine. Keep healing. Call on me for anything that you need.

Keep improvising. Keep adapting. Keep overcoming.

Text Messages: 10/11/12 11:15 AM

Carla: CeA in. 3.0 fucking awesome. Im in shock.

Me: That was quick. Holy fucking shit! Congratulations!

Me: You did it. You fucking did it.

Carla: Docs and nurses pretty blown away.

Me: I bet. So am I. Need to update my chart!

Carla: I am so blown away. Even my hair is growing back in.

Carla: 3.0! I am still in shock at how far I've come.

Me: You deserve every bit of good feeling that is coming over you right now.

Me: 3!!!!!!!

Me: Now that I've had some time to reflect on things - THREE POINT ZERO. You rock.

Carla: It's a miracle. Thank you for helping make this happen.

Me: It was always about your strength and your will. You have always been stronger than you realize. I am so proud and happy for you.

Me: You had a lot of support, but remember this - you did it. You lived through a lifetime of 3 AM moments.

Me: You gutted it out by yourself.

Me: You believed by yourself.

Me: And you won.

Me: I don't want to take away from your support team, but you won this. You lived it, and you deserve to be recognized as the winner.

Carla: No it took a whole team to keep me going and you were a part of that. Thank you my friend.

10/15/12 - Letter to Family / Friends

Inigo Montoya in The Princess Bride: No, there is too much. Let me sum up.

There is a theory of storytelling that dictates waiting until the last minute for the big reveal.

I do not subscribe to that theory. Carla's final marker number is 3. (Anything below 5 is considered to be cancer-free). The previous number was 4.2 - She is now free.

Anyone who might be offended by the profligate use of words that the FCC does not approve of would be well-advised to avert their eyes now.

She did it. She fucking did it. She was told that she had a 5% chance of living 4 months. My best friend blew right through that prognosis. This is the most awesomest thing ever.

Hollywood in Top Gun: Gutsiest move I ever saw, man.

I really don't know how to thank each of you for your help - each of you played a role, from Chad helping me to search for a stuffed turtle to Johnny II providing medical info to Bridget looping in her friends to help spread the load. I really don't want to leave anyone out - you were all invaluable.

You each helped to save someone's life, and for that I cannot possibly express my gratitude deeply enough.

And so I simply say thank you.

Carla and I had a great conversation last week. The summary, from someone who has looked into the abyss (her, not me), is this: DON'T WAIT. If there is something that you want to do, do it. I am fully aware that this concept is not anything new to most of you, but it is for me. Call it a reinforcement of things you already knew. Go out there. Do stuff. Do not have regrets.

Once again, Thank You.

Text Messages: 10/19/12 11:22 PM

Me: Have been thinking about something a lot lately - is there anything I can provide (mental / physical / emotional) that will make things easier for you? Don't be bashful.

Carla: I wish I could think of something but nothing comes to mind. Thanks for the offer. I am really feeling depressed just trying to get through this.

Me: Remember what you've overcome. Remember what you've done. Remember how strong you've shown yourself to be. You can get past this.

Carla: I know.

Text Messages: 10/22/12 11:12 PM

Me: Haven't forgotten about you. I think and worry about you constantly. Hope that you are doing ok.

Me: I love you more than you can possibly imagine - keep improvising, keep adapting, keep overcoming.

Carla: Well as things would have it im not so good. I am battling two bsd indections. Lot of pain and discofort. I hate this so much.

Text Messages: 10/28/12 11:58 AM

Carla: Thanks again for everything last night it was so fun. Miss hanging out with you so much. And thanks for getting me coffee this morning. I so appreciate it.

Me: It was so good to just laugh. Really enjoyed myself. Thanks for having me over.

November

Text Messages: 11/1/12 10:24 PM

Me: Checking in and hoping you are doing ok. Let me know if you need anything.

Carla: Not okay st all. Really sick from invections. Not getting bettet yet.

Text Messages: 11/3/12 3:43 PM

Carla: I dont knowv how you spent your Sat morning, but here is how I spent mine. Just had a home nurse input a catheter into my bladder. I get to wear this fall fashiong accessory for at least two weeks. Best part was that my mom assisted during the procedure. How is your weekend starting off. Sorry for all the sarcasm I am feeling sorry for myself.

Me: Don't be sorry. Ever. You are a survivor. You do what it takes. I am in awe of how powerful you are.

Me: In a different age, lyric poems would be written about you.

Me: You are a piece of iron. You are the strongest person I've ever known. You do the impossible.

Me: Stay strong. Stay true to who you are. Stay true to who you have always been. I love you more than you can possibly imagine.

Carla: If I'm so strong then why I can't stop crying.

Carla: I can't beat these things on my own. Lots of pressure on mom and Stu right now.

Me: Let me know if I can help in any way. I love you, and I think about ways to help you constantly.

Me: Stu and your mom are awesome. They are rocks for you to lean on. I'm very happy to know that you have them.

Me: I hope things are improving for you.

Carla: They are barley holging up.

Me: I'm thinking about you all the time. If you need anything, let me know.

Carla: Things are not improving and i'm starting to get scared.why is this happening. And why won't it get better.

Me: You will get better. Trust in that. Believe in that.

Text Messages: 11/9/12 5:29 PM

Me: I hope that you're feeling better and that your condition is improving.

Carla: No im very sick.

Me: Ok. Let me know if there is anything I can do for you or Stu.

Carla: Can you help me tomorrow night.

Me: Whatever you need.

Carla: I need someone to stay monday and Tuesday.

Me: I will be there.

11/11/12 Hi –

I guess I'm writing to tell you how I feel about you. I want you to know how deeply I value our friendship, and how it has matured over the years. I also want you to know how much I respect Stu for how he has both completed you and supported you. It was not by any means easy over the last couple of years, but you have both proven how much you belong together. I am equally awed and envious.

But this is not about me. This is about you. This is about reminding you that you are a survivor. You took the worst prognosis and you beat it. Because you could. Because of who you are. Because of your nature.

But you aren't just a survivor. You never have been. You are a conqueror. You didn't survive Wayne. You conquered him. You didn't survive Darren. You conquered him. I could continue the litany of things/people/situations, but there is no need to belabor the point. After a while, it becomes repetitive.

But with that repetition comes a theme. You do not give in. You may retreat, but that is tactical in nature, not strategic. Your 2012 has only been the latest manifestation of who you are.

I want you to know that I believe in you, Carla. I want to remind you of how strong you have been, and how strong you can be, regardless of how you feel. I want to remind you that you will win, because that is who you are, and that is who you have always been.

It seems a little trite to say it, but get well soon. We all want you back.

I love you more than you can possibly imagine.

11/11/12 - Stay Strong

After talking to you today, I know that you are worried and I know that you aren't sure what is going on. I don't have any answers for you right now.

What I do have is my love and support. What I do have is my knowledge of Stu's love and support. Your mom and a cast of hundreds stand by to try to help. I have watched and been awed by the number and variety of people who want to step up and help with your care.

We are all here for you. We want nothing less than for you to recover completely, and we are going to do everything we can to help make that happen.

Between The Naturopath and your other docs and your friends and your family, we will get you through this. Keep believing.

I will see you Monday night. If you need anything between then and now, please call/text/write. In the meantime, please keep believing. You are the strongest person I've ever known. You can finish this.

I love you more than you can possibly imagine.

11/15/12 - A quick note

I've been involved in an email exchange with my sisters about Alice's Christmas gift, and something struck me. I've learned that when I get these flashes, THEY ARE NOT COINCIDENCES.

Anyway, Bridget has been emailing from her work account. She works for Gold's Gym, and their motto is "know your own strength".

First, of course, it seems like you're pretty clear on that particular subject. But there is a secondary meaning that I am having a difficult time putting my finger on. It comes down to this, I think - you have proven to be stronger than you ever imagined yourself to be.

You are my best friend. I have loved every minute of the time we've spent together this year. The conversations we have had, typified by Tuesday night's discussions, have been so much fun.

I guess I just want you to know that we are going to have a lot more of them, and in far better circumstances. The Naturopath was right back in June when he told me that you would be laughing about this two years from now. Everything is in place to give you a full recovery. There will soon be a path forward, and then you can finally put this in your past and go on to be the best Carla that you can be.

I love you more than you can possibly imagine. Please let me know if you need anything.

11/16/12 - Letter to Family / Friends

I don't have all the details, and won't until after I see her tonight, but it is back. Her CEA number post-chemo has jumped from 3 to 21, and her docs have told her that the only thing that they can do is give her more chemo treatments. She made the decision a long time ago that she was only going to go the chemo route once, and she's decided to stick with that choice.

We saved her, and it is all going to be for nothing. All the pain that she endured, all the three AM moments. Everything.

I'm pretty much numb at this point and words are not coming easily, but I wanted to let everyone know and to say thanks for all that you did for her and for me.

11/17/12 - Letter to Family / Friends

I went to see Carla today at the hospital. A fast-growing tumor has invaded her bladder and her kidneys. It is about the size of her fist. She'll be having a procedure where they reroute the kidney output to a bag rather than through the urethra, which is basically closed off due to the tumor.

The best guess is 3-4 weeks or so left.

For all of that, she is in wonderful spirits. She's very calm and peaceful and almost happy. There was no crying or pain - just laughter. We talked about what we have meant to each other over the years. We talked about great memories. She is at peace and ready to move on with zero regrets, which is the best that any of us can expect or hope for.

11/19/12 - The Talk We Had

(After the bad news that there was a new tumor, and that it wasn't really treatable, and that Carla only had a limited time left, I spent a lot of time at her house watching her dogs (and mine) while Stu was at the hospital. I was able to spend a lot of time with Carla during the days, and I wrote her one last letter, which I read to her in person. This was both the most difficult and easiest thing I've ever done.)

So, I'm sitting downstairs right now watching the Steelers game and hanging out with the dogs. The house is empty and quiet.

I'm thinking about all of the wonderful times we had in this basement and about the fact that Thanksgiving is coming up and that next year I won't be able to share Thanksgiving with you.

I'm trying to be as strong as I can for you, and I am breathing like you told me to do, but it is moments like this that hit me hard, when I reflect on what it is going to be like without you in my life.

My Aunt Kazuko and I have had a long-running email conversation since January about a lot of things, but mainly about you. She said today that she is really most upset about the fact that she isn't going to get a chance to know you.

Here is a direct quote from my response to her:

"I remember very clearly the night that Fox passed away - Carla took me out for drinks before my redeye back to Pittsburgh, and she told me that she wished that she had met him. I told her that he was so much a part of me that she already had. The same applies here - you've already met her and gotten to know her."

I know you will always be a part of me, and I just want you to know how incredibly important you have been to me, and how many things you've taught me and continue to teach me.

I understand that you are taking the next step, and the way you described things getting wavy is of tremendous comfort to me. I'm not scared any more, and I hope you aren't either.

I love you Carla, more than anyone I've ever known. I'm going to miss you more than I can possibly imagine, but I know now that this is not the end, that there is so much more to look forward to. You are my best friend, and I am forever changed because of who you are.

(When I was done, Carla laid in the bed for a moment or two, her eyes closed. She opened them, looked at me, and said "how can I be sad if someone writes something like that about me? I must have done something right.")

11/20/12 - Memorial Party Invite First Draft

I've been working on the email that we are going to send out. This is what I've come up with so far. It needs a lot of revisions, but I've tried to adhere to the spirit of our conversations, and I've tried to adopt your voice as best I can.

I will see you on Sunday and we can talk about changes that you want.

Love you!

We're having a memorial service for Carla on xxxxxx date at Fado in Seattle. Doors open at xxxx.

Carla asked specifically for several things:

1) No speeches. First, because most of them will be lame (direct quote). Second, because she could out-talk all of you. This is also a direct quote. You come at the Queen, you'd best not miss.

2) No drama. This rule will be strictly enforced by her roving band of, um, Enforcers. There is too much in life to be distracted by petty bullshit. Again, this rule comes directly from Carla - she is watching to make sure you comply.

3) No flowers. We quote Carla directly: "yuck". If you feel the need to spend money, (and you should) please donate it to Noel House. Or donate some canned goods to your local shelter. One of her biggest passions was feeding people, and it pissed her off that in a country as rich as ours people are starving. Seriously. Help, even if you only do it for a week. Then do it for another week until it becomes a habit.

4) Have fun. This isn't about loss. This is about celebrating a life well lived, and without regrets, because she didn't have any.

5) Go forth and apply what she learned:

- Make the world better.

- Feed people, whether with actual food or wisdom/spirituality.

- Seriously, no speeches. You are collectively bad at that part.

- Dave Matthews tells us that life is short and sweet, but certain. Resolve the petty bullshit now and put it in your past. Leave it there.

11/20/12 - Letter to Family / Friends

Apologies in advance - this is a long one, even by my standards. I am writing this from the C&S Lounge, which is the name that we bestowed upon the basement bar that Stu and Carla installed about 5 minutes after they moved into their house. It is a full, and I do mean full, bar.

For the last 11-1/2 months, it was also often where I would go, after Carla went to sleep. I would get drunk and write her emails to try to keep her going, to keep her inspired. I would write to keep myself inspired in the face of anxiety and horror and uncertainty. She always said that she could tell when I was stressed, even before all of this happened, because she would receive a 4,000 word rant, (produced with no typos on an iPhone (her words, but a source of personal pride)) in her email on the way to work. My best guess is that I've written over 60,000 words to her this year. A typical book comes in at about 35,000.

I wrote my final email to her two nights ago, and the funny thing is that I didn't really say anything that I haven't said a zillion times before. I read it to her in the hospital last night, rather than just zapping it off, which seemed a little impersonal. It was simultaneously the easiest and most difficult thing I've ever done. I choked my way through it, and at the end she had nothing but smiles. This is not a time for sadness; this is a time for celebration of a life lived well.

She is comfortable with the life that she has led and the fact that she's done everything she wanted to do. There are no regrets at all.

From here on out, I've resolved not to talk to her of sickness or cancer or illness. Now it is just about enjoying each other, as we have since April 1999, when we first met at a business function.

She's home from the hospital now, and a lot more comfortable. The kidney reroute was successful, and they did a nerve block (still don't know what this is, but it sounds cool) in her pelvis, so she won't feel any more pain.

I spent a lot of time with her this weekend. Most of it was watching her sleep. After nearly a year of watching her sleep, I can tell that something has changed in her breathing rhythm. Her voice, the most truly distinctive part of her personality - something that would fill any room she was in, has gotten a lot quieter. The time is growing near.

But for all of that, for how quickly things have reversed themselves, she is unbelievably calm and relaxed. She told me that she is comfortable that she did everything she could, and now is the time to prepare to move on. She's made peace with it, as well as with the people in her life.

She did tell me about something extraordinary that happened on Saturday night. She was just laying there, watching some mindless TV show, and the room started to get all wavy, as she describes it. She could feel herself being enveloped by the waves, and she had a choice to make about whether or not to stay.

Obviously, she decided not to go yet, but the fact that she had a choice is tremendously comforting. The provenance of this story is important. Carla's my best friend. As she and I used to say, there are friends who help you move, and there are friends who help you move bodies. The distinction is subtle but important. I have always trusted her implicitly.

Her experience is as close as I will come (until I experience it myself) of a world larger than what we see and experience every day. As someone who has not been particularly spiritual in my life (other than the retail-level philosophy dispensed by George Lucas in Episodes IV-VI, episodes I-III HAVING NEVER EXISTED), this was an awakening for me. She's taught me one last thing.

In the movie Signs, there is a critical moment where Mel Gibson's character talks about coincidences, and the fact that there are two types of people in the world - those that see them and those that don't. I am comforted, after this experience, that I am one of those who sees them. I don't know what this means for me going forward, whether I will turn to Jesus or Vishnu or Allah or Buddha, but I know now that there is something larger and more wonderful than I can ever imagine.

More than living up to some figurehead for a religion, though, I want to live up to what Carla told me, shortly after being told that the end is coming soon - "I've had a great life. I've done everything I wanted to. I've had great relationships. I have zero regrets. What else could you ask for?"

The Naturopath talks, on a regular basis, about the fact that we will all die eventually. We are born, we live, and we die. At the end, we have the story of our life. It is up to us to have a good story to tell. Carla is fortunate in that she does. It is up to the rest of us to learn from her example.

IN CASE I AM BEING TOO SUBTLE: DON'T LEAVE ANYTHING IN THE LOCKER ROOM. LIVE YOUR LIFE WELL AND HAVE ZERO REGRETS.

As a practical matter, it is likely that I will not send another one of these emails until after Carla has passed away. They are difficult to write, and I anticipate that hearing about the mechanics of the final steps will be more than you all want to get with your morning coffee. If you want to hear details as things come to pass, please let me know.

Finally, thank you all for letting me send this stuff out on a regular basis. You have no idea how much easier it made things, and I thank all of you.

Text Messages: 11/25/12 10:45 PM

Me: Carla, I love you and I am praying for you. May you be bathed in Light.

Carla: Thank you. The past two days have been very difficult but thankyou for staying. I am feeling sllghtly better. Pleasse keep up the good thoughts and prayers. Lovr you honey.

11/26/12 - Letter to Family / Friends

"I need you to breathe for me, honey."

That's what she told me to do. She didn't want me to cry. She wanted me to accept, as she had, the inevitable.

There, two Fridays ago, while sitting on the concrete steps outside of the office, I listened as she laid out the truth. Her CEA number had jumped from 3 to 21. The biopsy had come back lousy with cancer cells. She was on the way to the hospital.

I remember very few things about that conversation. She was crying a little and difficult to understand. Plus my head and heart were in the process of melting down. But I do remember her telling me to breathe.

I've moved, I think, into acceptance, although every so often the fact that we won't meet after work for too many drinks is not going to happen again in this life rears its ugly head, and I am unspeakably shaken to my core.

But here's the thing. I must speak of it. I must speak of how, moments after she found out that she was going to die, and soon, one of her first thoughts was to call me and tell me to breathe. What an amazing person, and how fortunate I am to have known her.

In The Art of Racing in the Rain, the story is told from the point of view of the family dog. The first line is "large gestures are all that I have." While I've always had a gift for putting the noun and the verb in the right place, I have not ever been the most spiritually or emotionally open person that you know, so all of the things that I speak of, all of this stuff, feels like I'm painting with a fire hose when a tiny brush would be far more effective. All I have is large gestures, and they will have to suffice.

One of my favorite authors, Neal Stephenson, had an on-point observation about what is coming in his book Reamde: "Each death meant that a particular set of perceptions and reactions was gone from the world, apparently forever, and served as a reminder to Richard that one day his ideas and perceptions would be gone too."

We can argue about the mechanics of this, about what happens to the spirit after it separates from the body, but the simple fact is that we Don't Know.

I disagree with Stephenson on one point - I believe that after the spirit and the body are separated, the spirit lives on. Energy can neither be created nor destroyed. This is an immutable law of physics as we understand it, and I'm enough of a science geek that it makes sense to me.

And so I did what she told me to do. I breathed. In between bouts of crying, of course.

I can't imagine a world where her perceptions and reactions are not instantly accessible, where I can't call her up just to say hi and get involved in a thirty-minute conversation that hits on politics and human rights and movies and the Seahawks and pop culture and literature and the inherent deficiencies of soccer. This, I think, is going to suck. A lot.

She is sleeping enough to make my dog jealous now - hard not to when you're on 20 mg of Oxycodone every 4 hours. The likelihood that she and I will have another conversation of any meaning is improbably low. I'm lucky in that I had the two days in the hospital with her, when she was pretty coherent, and we were able to connect one last time. I asked her if she really was as calm as she seemed, and I told her to tell me the truth. Yes, she told me, I'm unbelievably calm, and not just trying to be strong for people around me.

The best part, aside from knowing and feeling her acceptance, is that there was nothing unresolved between us, no settling of accounts. I think I'm happiest about that fact, that we didn't have any regrets or lingering crap to deal with. Nothing but joy about a life well lived.

I know I'm late to the party on the whole spirituality and prayer thing. Too much Roman Catholicism, I suppose. Through this disaster I have discovered something a bit more subtle than a God who says, in the words of Dogma, one of my favorite movies, "Do what I tell you to do or I'm going to fucking spank you."

I found a book by Anne Lamott that I highly recommend, called Help. Thanks. Wow. (Her definition of the three types of prayer, separated from all of the religious BS that has grown up around some really basic ideas). She has a really simple prayer (from the Help chapter) that she uses in situations like this, and it appealed to me enough that I'm going to pass it along - "Please Bathe her in Your Light and Peace. Amen."

And now we wait, and try to breathe. Thanks to all for helping me shoulder this.

11/28/12 - Letter to Family / Friends

Yes, I know. Things have not looked good recently. And the overall trend is down. This is also not good.

You know what is good? Morphine drips. At least to the extent that she's not feeling a whole lot of pain right now.

Let's set aside the whole reason for why she's in this position, that her days are numbered. For the first time in 12 months, she is feeling no pain.

I went to the house tonight expecting more of the same - watching her sleep and asking for her to be bathed in light and comfort. Instead, I got a very welcome surprise in the form of a text message as I drove up:

"Looking forward to seeing you. Please please bring ne a can of cocke. J ust a can and dont bring it out until he is gone. Besides he is so happy that I ate a real meal today he will let me have anything today!"

Spelling was never her strong suit, but I love her anyway. Stu docsn't want her to have sugar as it feeds the tumors; I have been her Coca-Cola dealer since the terminal diagnosis, because it makes her happy and it really doesn't matter any more. Yes, I verified this with the hospice nurse. I LOVE being her coke dealer, so to speak.

After yesterday's email, you would reasonably expect more documentation of the slow spiral downward. Not tonight.

She was alert and funny and...Carla. Now that she doesn't have to deal with pain on a regular basis, she can be herself again. I have no idea how long this is going to last, but tonight felt like a gift. Let me repeat that, because it is important. Tonight was a gift for me. I did not expect that I'd be able to interact with her like this again.

We talked about 13 years of memories, and I held her hand. She kept squeezing mine. I assumed that she was hurting, as that had been our signal. No, she explained - that's her system for remembering things - as people visit her, she grabs their hands, and as things from the past wash over her, she squeezes the hand to try to imprint it on her spirit, to carry it over in some way.

Suffice it to say, we've had a lot of amazing memories, and her grip is as strong as it has ever been.

We talked about everything from pop culture (she still has a weakness for pop culture, and the latest 2-1/2 Men controversy fascinated her) to politics to sports.

It was 3 glorious hours. There were a few minutes of pathos, as you might expect, but my overwhelming feeling tonight as I left was one of joy, of being given another chance to hang out with my best friend.

I talked yesterday of the three basic prayers - Help, Thanks, Wow. As I was driving home tonight, I experienced all three almost simultaneously: Help my friend by bathing her in Light, Thanks for giving me another chance to talk to her; Wow, I was lucky enough to connect with her for as long as I did. Humbling.

As we draw closer to the point where she isn't physically tangible, I recognize how much I will miss her. At the same time, it really is going to be OK, and I know that now.

Tonight was a gift for me, one that I recognized immediately. It was a pleasure to hold her hand and talk of memories. I know her time is measured in days or weeks. I don't want to get too deep or morbid, but I'm sure that in your lives there are people that you care deeply about.

LET THEM KNOW THAT YOU DO.

If I've learned anything through this process, it is that we assume things will always be a certain way and are utterly unprepared when things go a different way. It will happen; this is the human condition.

I thank all of you for listening to me and helping me to share the burden.

December

A Final Text Message From The Big C

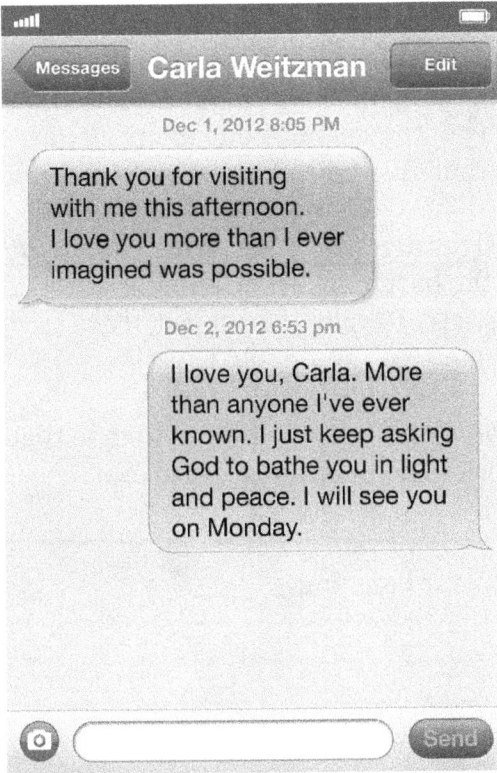

Carla Weitzman

Dec 1, 2012 8:05 PM

Thank you for visiting with me this afternoon. I love you more than I ever imagined was possible.

Dec 2, 2012 6:53 pm

I love you, Carla. More than anyone I've ever known. I just keep asking God to bathe you in light and peace. I will see you on Monday.

12/11/12 - Letter to Family / Friends

Stu invited a small group of Carla's friends over on Monday night as a way for all of us to say goodbye, one and two at a time. I spent my time reciting Hail Mary's (badly - I kept skipping entire sections due to my 20 year lapse from being a Catholic).

He is being enormously protective of her, which I approve of heartily. We sat in the basement of the house and toasted her at great length. Despite the subject, there were only smiles and laughter, as we told Carla stories.

I can't think of a better legacy to try to live up to than that. I also have a lot of work to do in order to get to that minimum standard.

As always, thanks to all for listening.

The Actual Worst Text Message of All Time

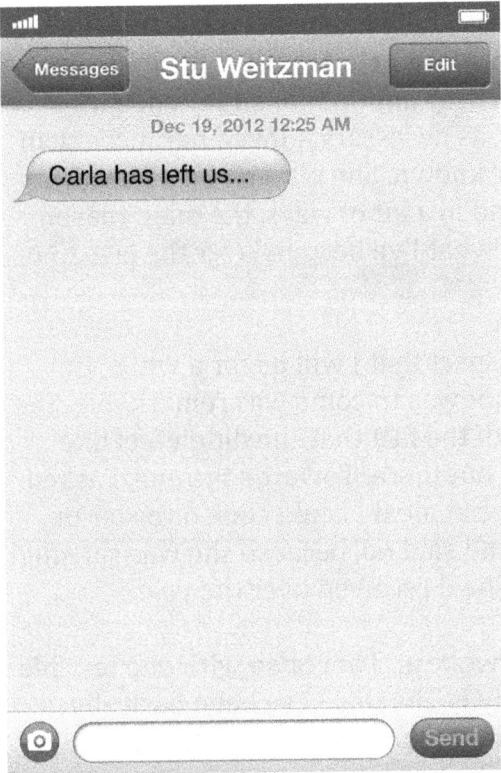

12/19/12 - Letter to Family / Friends

Carla passed away peacefully in her sleep last night. I will miss her tremendously, but I suspect that she'll be around for a while, in one form or another, to either encourage me or to kick my ass, as necessary. I loved her more than anyone that I've ever known. She was my best friend, my motivator in chief, and in a lot of ways, the main reason why I've turned into what I've become over the last 13 or 14 years.

Yes, I'm sad, and I suspect that I will be for a while. But her acceptance of what was to come was remarkable. She was especially ok with the fact that she didn't feel like she'd left a whole lot out there. Towards the end, I asked her if there was a special meal I could cook or order in, and she just smiled and said no, because she was satisfied with the things that she'd received over the years.

All week last week, I woke at 3 am or so with one terrible thought: What if today is The Day? I've been basically useless (or more useless than usual) at work as a result, as that question reverberated through my head.

Once again, The Naturopath stepped into the breach on Thursday afternoon. I was describing the 3 am moments, and he asked, "What if today was The Day for you, not for Carla?" My first flippant comment was that I'd probably be found in the candy aisle at Safeway, making up for 12 years of lost sugar consumption.

That isn't a way to live, though, and I get The Naturopath's more subtle point - when I woke up this morning, the question on my mind was this - "what is the most important thing I can do today?" The answer is going to vary by the day or by the hour, of course. It would be nice to live in a state where there were no

398

consequences, to be freed from long-term concerns, and to simply enjoy.

That isn't realistic, of course. There are "addictions to pay and bills to feed," to quote Jewel (Carla would kick my ass if she knew I was quoting Jewel, but whatever - sometimes the ends justify the means). Just to prove that 12 years of Catholic education wasn't completely wasted, I'll weave in something Biblical with a similar meaning: "Give to Caesar what is Caesar's." Jesus may have been a really good carpenter and an award-winning cook on Top Chef with his loaves and fishes topped with garlic butter (I look at food with garlic butter on/in it primarily as a means of conveying more garlic butter onto my tongue and into my stomach) as well as the greatest bartender of all time, but the mortgage still needs to be paid, and the dog fed, and the kids hugged.

Look - I know I'm the last person to be talking about this stuff - my spiritual tank has been on empty for a long time before this all started, and you can probably chalk some of this up to stress and grief. The simple logical question remains, however: What If?

Most of all, I'll remember her laugh. Whether the subject was serious or silly, she found a way to laugh about it, to see through the stupidity. I think, most of all, that I will miss that the most.

Farewell Carla, and Godspeed.

Epilogue

Well, that was not the result that I had been hoping and praying for throughout the entirety of 2012. I often wish that there had been a happier end to the story, that everything that Carla had done, and all of her friends and family had done for her, would have paid off in the way that we all wanted it to.

In the end, though, that was not to be. Looking back, she had been living on borrowed time ever since that first diagnosis in early January; Herman was 15 centimeters (almost 6 inches) and while we could forestall the outcome, I've really come to understand that it was always going to play out this way. I think that deep down she knew what was going to happen, and that's why when the news finally came down she was so calm about it - she had been coming to terms with it for nearly 12 months.

I am proud, of course, that I was there to stand up for her, to remind her that I didn't want to see her fail, and I was going to do whatever I could to ensure that she was going to not just survive, but thrive.

At the same time, I'm horrified at a stat that The Naturopath told me somewhere along the way - the cancer rate in 1900 was roughly 1 in 100 - for his age group, it is approaching 1 in 2. Carla was 45 when she was diagnosed, 5 years before the docs even recommend testing for colon cancer. The number of younger people who are being diagnosed with all forms of cancer is one of the underreported statistics of our age. While studies vary, I wonder how much of this can be correlated with the massive amount of toxins we ingest in our daily lives. I know I'm not a doc, just some guy who lost his best friend to a disease that she shouldn't have gotten in the first place, but we have to start rolling this shit back or it will consume us.

The Naturopath, as I've pointed out, keeps telling me that there are some immutable truths - we are born, we live, and then we all die. In between, we tell our story - it is really the only thing we leave behind when we're gone. Carla left a great story behind when she died. This single year was only a part of it. She was an absolutely remarkable woman, even though you didn't hear a lot from her in this book. The number of people that she touched, not just on a professional level, but, more importantly, on a personal level, was evident in the number of people who tried to help out through the ordeal.

This story, however, takes two to tango. The Chris Sypolt writing to Carla in late January is not the same one who penned the final message that I read to her in her hospital room in November. I am irrevocably changed (mostly for the better) by this experience, although I would have preferred that it didn't happen for another 30 years or so. I miss my friend, sometimes desperately, but I am comforted by the memories that she and I shared, not just during 2012, but in all the years that we had before. It is remarkable, looking back, just how easy it was to write many of these emails - this was just a single-minded commitment to helping my friend in whatever way I could and, in many ways, as only I could do for her. The Muses definitely helped.

That, and scotch. Lots and lots of scotch.

In December of 2000, my dad (The Fox) passed away due to complications from emphysema. Carla took me out for drinks the night that it happened - I was booked on a redeye back to Pittsburgh that night and needed to kill some time. We had a lot of drinks, even for us, and somehow got on the subject of the three songs that we wanted to be played at our funerals. We wrote them

402

down on the back of a business card and promised that we would always carry them.

Here were Carla's:

1. American Girl by Tom Petty & the Heartbreakers. On our second date, way back in 1999, we ended up sitting on her front porch and drinking hefeweizen on a perfect Seattle summer afternoon. American Girl came on the radio, and we ended up dancing on her front lawn. Just an amazing memory that we both shared.

2. Two Step by the Dave Matthews Band - it happened to be playing that night on the jukebox, and she seized upon it. There is one line that jumped out to her: "Life is short and sweet but certain." There was no way, on that cold December night, that we could know just how true that statement would turn out to be.

3. Into The Mystic by Van Morrison - I'm not even going to try to explain how appropriate that song was. It still tears my guts out every time I hear it.

Carla was very specific with her last wishes, and told Stu early on in their relationship about the existence of the list. He was able to find a musician to play at her memorial party who could cover the songs. As the opening notes of Into The Mystic started to play, I pulled out the business card that I had been carrying for the past dozen or so years and wept openly as my final goodbye to her played out. It was ultimately cathartic - Carla was indeed going home, and at some level, at least, I had helped to make the transition as easy as I possibly could for her. My duty to her had come to an end. I kept the business card, though, and eventually found an appropriate place for it.

There is nothing ultimately redemptive about cancer. It is, after all, just one more way that we come to our end. The nature of it, the slow, inexorable erosion, however, leaves us with plenty of time to think and to reflect on the people we are and who we hoped to become. I loved Carla with all of my heart, and in the end, it wasn't enough. But in all of our conversations, in the things that were said, as well as the ones that weren't said, there was never any doubt in our minds that we had made a very deep connection, and that we were lucky to have each other, no matter how short that time was. In her struggle, I found a new lens to look at life. I will remember that forever.

My friend Marianne, who was kind enough to write the Foreword, sees Letters To The Big C in a different light. Marianne has survived cancer. It cost her a lung, and her ability to travel in an airplane, amongst other things. She sees Letters as me providing armor that Carla could put on every day. I don't know what the right answer is. I do know that I am forever changed by having been part of Carla's life and having the honor to help her in her darkest hours.

This, then, is the lesson that I learned. Be present for the people in your life, not just when they are going through something serious, but when everything is going well. Use whatever gifts you have to help the ones around you. Don't be a fatalist, but remember that every day might be The Day. Make choices that honor this fact. If you've made mistakes up to this point, it isn't too late to make things right, to show your emotions and feelings and love. Life is too short to spend it on irrelevant bullshit.

Above all, decide what your story is going to be, no matter what form it takes, and get busy telling it.

Chris Sypolt
Seattle, WA, October 2013

Acknowledgements

First of all, I want to thank Carla's husband, Stu Weitzman, for his gracious permission to use Carla's words (mainly her text messages) in telling this story. It wouldn't have been nearly as effective without hearing some of her words. We are donating 10% of the proceeds of this thing to cancer-related charities, and we both thank you for your help.

(Stu was also kind enough to provide the picture of all of three of us that I used at the beginning of the book. Here's another one, from a happier afternoon.)

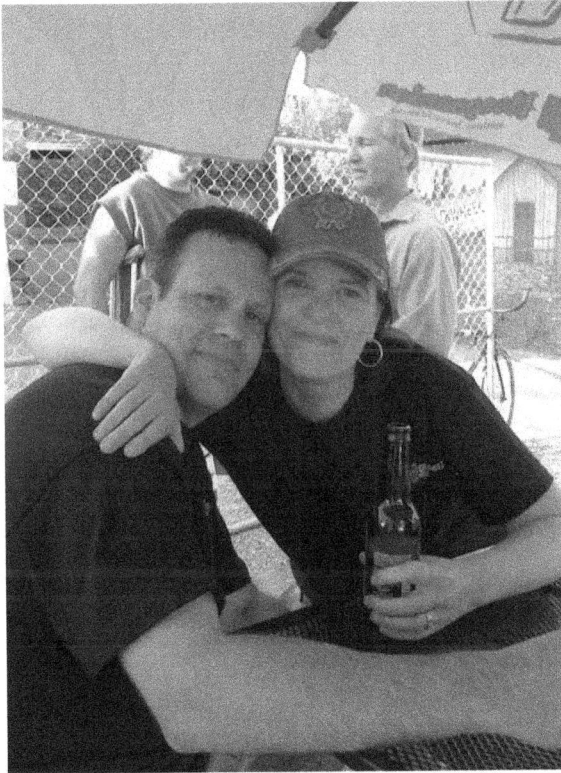

Second, to my family and friends, who were the recipients of many of the emails I sent out, and who were so kind and helpful with their tolerance of my ranting, as well as making helpful suggestions. I hate singling out any one person, because they all did their part, but my Aunt Kazuko really stood out, not just because she listened, but if I had gone too long without reporting in, she was always the first one to check in with me.

Third, for the small army of volunteer editors that I pressed into service to help me, chief amongst them my sister Bridget and my very close friend Marianne (who wrote the foreword) - both provided incredibly valuable insight into some of the things that worked, and some that didn't, even though I didn't take a lot of their advice.

I want to thank all of my friends and coworkers at OnlineMetals, who took over a lot of the load when I was off running errands or doing hospital pickups or, especially towards the end, when I was simply inconsolable and unable to do my job properly.

Just because I am, at the end of the day, a ridiculous geek, I'd also like to say thank you to the creators of SimpleNote. I wrote virtually every word of the letters to Carla using their simple, yet enormously powerful, iPhone app.

I'd like to thank all of my bartenders, in no particular order, who kept my morose ass in scotch throughout the year. You provided the fuel that I needed to write this stuff in the first place: Brad, Jeremy, Makenna, Brandi Jean, Sheena, the other Brandi, Robin, and probably a dozen others whose names are slipping my mind, including the entire staff of the Royal Lahaina hotel in Maui, where I spent two blissful weeks in the beginning of May 2013 attempting to put myself together after Carla's passing.

But it would take a whole other book to tell that story.

About the Author

Chris Sypolt grew up in Pittsburgh, PA, and now lives in Seattle with his dog BJ, where they have had a running 10 year contest over who can be better at napping, eating, and then napping again. The dog, unencumbered by a job or career, has a nearly insurmountable lead in this game, but that hasn't stopped Chris from attempting to catch up.

Do not make the mistake of claiming that Armageddon is a bad movie around him. He owns the Director's Cut.

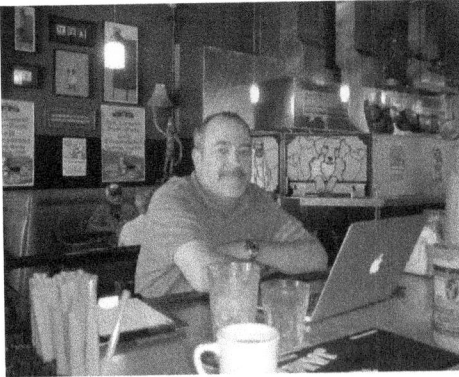

He can be found on Twitter with a username of @cdsypolt.

Letters To The Big C is his first book.